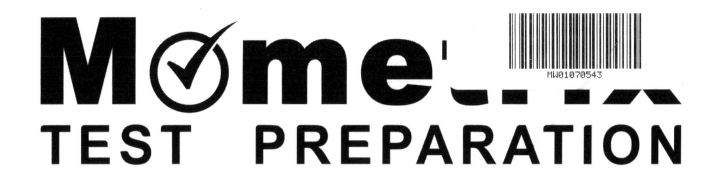

AOCNP®

Exam Secrets
Study Guide
Part 1 of 2

DEAR FUTURE EXAM SUCCESS STORY

First of all, **THANK YOU** for purchasing Mometrix study materials!

Second, congratulations! You are one of the few determined test-takers who are committed to doing whatever it takes to excel on your exam. **You have come to the right place.** We developed these study materials with one goal in mind: to deliver you the information you need in a format that's concise and easy to use.

In addition to optimizing your guide for the content of the test, we've outlined our recommended steps for breaking down the preparation process into small, attainable goals so you can make sure you stay on track.

We've also analyzed the entire test-taking process, identifying the most common pitfalls and showing how you can overcome them and be ready for any curveball the test throws you.

Standardized testing is one of the biggest obstacles on your road to success, which only increases the importance of doing well in the high-pressure, high-stakes environment of test day. Your results on this test could have a significant impact on your future, and this guide provides the information and practical advice to help you achieve your full potential on test day.

Your success is our success

We would love to hear from you! If you would like to share the story of your exam success or if you have any questions or comments in regard to our products, please contact us at **800-673-8175** or **support@mometrix.com**.

Thanks again for your business and we wish you continued success!

Sincerely,
The Mometrix Test Preparation Team

> **Need more help? Check out our flashcards at:**
> **http://mometrixflashcards.com/ONCC**

TABLE OF CONTENTS

Introduction

Thank you for purchasing this resource! You have made the choice to prepare yourself for a test that could have a huge impact on your future, and this guide is designed to help you be fully ready for test day. Obviously, it's important to have a solid understanding of the test material, but you also need to be prepared for the unique environment and stressors of the test, so that you can perform to the best of your abilities.

For this purpose, the first section that appears in this guide is the **Secret Keys**. We've devoted countless hours to meticulously researching what works and what doesn't, and we've boiled down our findings to the five most impactful steps you can take to improve your performance on the test. We start at the beginning with study planning and move through the preparation process, all the way to the testing strategies that will help you get the most out of what you know when you're finally sitting in front of the test.

We recommend that you start preparing for your test as far in advance as possible. However, if you've bought this guide as a last-minute study resource and only have a few days before your test, we recommend that you skip over the first two Secret Keys since they address a long-term study plan.

If you struggle with **test anxiety**, we strongly encourage you to check out our recommendations for how you can overcome it. Test anxiety is a formidable foe, but it can be beaten, and we want to make sure you have the tools you need to defeat it.

1

Secret Key #1 – Plan Big, Study Small

There's a lot riding on your performance. If you want to ace this test, you're going to need to keep your skills sharp and the material fresh in your mind. You need a plan that lets you review everything you need to know while still fitting in your schedule. We'll break this strategy down into three categories.

Information Organization

Start with the information you already have: the official test outline. From this, you can make a complete list of all the concepts you need to cover before the test. Organize these concepts into groups that can be studied together, and create a list of any related vocabulary you need to learn so you can brush up on any difficult terms. You'll want to keep this vocabulary list handy once you actually start studying since you may need to add to it along the way.

Time Management

Once you have your set of study concepts, decide how to spread them out over the time you have left before the test. Break your study plan into small, clear goals so you have a manageable task for each day and know exactly what you're doing. Then just focus on one small step at a time. When you manage your time this way, you don't need to spend hours at a time studying. Studying a small block of content for a short period each day helps you retain information better and avoid stressing over how much you have left to do. You can relax knowing that you have a plan to cover everything in time. In order for this strategy to be effective though, you have to start studying early and stick to your schedule. Avoid the exhaustion and futility that comes from last-minute cramming!

Study Environment

The environment you study in has a big impact on your learning. Studying in a coffee shop, while probably more enjoyable, is not likely to be as fruitful as studying in a quiet room. It's important to keep distractions to a minimum. You're only planning to study for a short block of time, so make the most of it. Don't pause to check your phone or get up to find a snack. It's also important to **avoid multitasking**. Research has consistently shown that multitasking will make your studying dramatically less effective. Your study area should also be comfortable and well-lit so you don't have the distraction of straining your eyes or sitting on an uncomfortable chair.

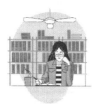 The time of day you study is also important. You want to be rested and alert. Don't wait until just before bedtime. Study when you'll be most likely to comprehend and remember. Even better, if you know what time of day your test will be, set that time aside for study. That way your brain will be used to working on that subject at that specific time and you'll have a better chance of recalling information.

Finally, it can be helpful to team up with others who are studying for the same test. Your actual studying should be done in as isolated an environment as possible, but the work of organizing the information and setting up the study plan can be divided up. In between study sessions, you can discuss with your teammates the concepts that you're all studying and quiz each other on the details. Just be sure that your teammates are as serious about the test as you are. If you find that your study time is being replaced with social time, you might need to find a new team.

2

Secret Key #2 – Make Your Studying Count

You're devoting a lot of time and effort to preparing for this test, so you want to be absolutely certain it will pay off. This means doing more than just reading the content and hoping you can remember it on test day. It's important to make every minute of study count. There are two main areas you can focus on to make your studying count.

Retention

It doesn't matter how much time you study if you can't remember the material. You need to make sure you are retaining the concepts. To check your retention of the information you're learning, try recalling it at later times with minimal prompting. Try carrying around flashcards and glance at one or two from time to time or ask a friend who's also studying for the test to quiz you.

To enhance your retention, look for ways to put the information into practice so that you can apply it rather than simply recalling it. If you're using the information in practical ways, it will be much easier to remember. Similarly, it helps to solidify a concept in your mind if you're not only reading it to yourself but also explaining it to someone else. Ask a friend to let you teach them about a concept you're a little shaky on (or speak aloud to an imaginary audience if necessary). As you try to summarize, define, give examples, and answer your friend's questions, you'll understand the concepts better and they will stay with you longer. Finally, step back for a big picture view and ask yourself how each piece of information fits with the whole subject. When you link the different concepts together and see them working together as a whole, it's easier to remember the individual components.

Finally, practice showing your work on any multi-step problems, even if you're just studying. Writing out each step you take to solve a problem will help solidify the process in your mind, and you'll be more likely to remember it during the test.

Modality

Modality simply refers to the means or method by which you study. Choosing a study modality that fits your own individual learning style is crucial. No two people learn best in exactly the same way, so it's important to know your strengths and use them to your advantage.

For example, if you learn best by visualization, focus on visualizing a concept in your mind and draw an image or a diagram. Try color-coding your notes, illustrating them, or creating symbols that will trigger your mind to recall a learned concept. If you learn best by hearing or discussing information, find a study partner who learns the same way or read aloud to yourself. Think about how to put the information in your own words. Imagine that you are giving a lecture on the topic and record yourself so you can listen to it later.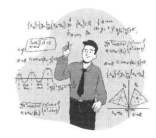

For any learning style, flashcards can be helpful. Organize the information so you can take advantage of spare moments to review. Underline key words or phrases. Use different colors for different categories. Mnemonic devices (such as creating a short list in which every item starts with the same letter) can also help with retention. Find what works best for you and use it to store the information in your mind most effectively and easily.

3

Secret Key #3 – Practice the Right Way

Your success on test day depends not only on how many hours you put into preparing, but also on whether you prepared the right way. It's good to check along the way to see if your studying is paying off. One of the most effective ways to do this is by taking practice tests to evaluate your progress. Practice tests are useful because they show exactly where you need to improve. Every time you take a practice test, pay special attention to these three groups of questions:

- The questions you got wrong
- The questions you had to guess on, even if you guessed right
- The questions you found difficult or slow to work through

This will show you exactly what your weak areas are, and where you need to devote more study time. Ask yourself why each of these questions gave you trouble. Was it because you didn't understand the material? Was it because you didn't remember the vocabulary? Do you need more repetitions on this type of question to build speed and confidence? Dig into those questions and figure out how you can strengthen your weak areas as you go back to review the material.

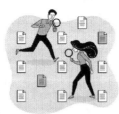 Additionally, many practice tests have a section explaining the answer choices. It can be tempting to read the explanation and think that you now have a good understanding of the concept. However, an explanation likely only covers part of the question's broader context. Even if the explanation makes perfect sense, **go back and investigate** every concept related to the question until you're positive you have a thorough understanding.

As you go along, keep in mind that the practice test is just that: practice. Memorizing these questions and answers will not be very helpful on the actual test because it is unlikely to have any of the same exact questions. If you only know the right answers to the sample questions, you won't be prepared for the real thing. **Study the concepts** until you understand them fully, and then you'll be able to answer any question that shows up on the test.

It's important to wait on the practice tests until you're ready. If you take a test on your first day of study, you may be overwhelmed by the amount of material covered and how much you need to learn. Work up to it gradually.

On test day, you'll need to be prepared for answering questions, managing your time, and using the test-taking strategies you've learned. It's a lot to balance, like a mental marathon that will have a big impact on your future. Like training for a marathon, you'll need to start slowly and work your way up. When test day arrives, you'll be ready.

Start with the strategies you've read in the first two Secret Keys—plan your course and study in the way that works best for you. If you have time, consider using multiple study resources to get different approaches to the same concepts. It can be helpful to see difficult concepts from more than one angle. Then find a good source for practice tests. Many times, the test website will suggest potential study resources or provide sample tests.

Practice Test Strategy

If you're able to find at least three practice tests, we recommend this strategy:

Untimed and Open-Book Practice

Take the first test with no time constraints and with your notes and study guide handy. Take your time and focus on applying the strategies you've learned.

Timed and Open-Book Practice

Take the second practice test open-book as well, but set a timer and practice pacing yourself to finish in time.

Timed and Closed-Book Practice

Take any other practice tests as if it were test day. Set a timer and put away your study materials. Sit at a table or desk in a quiet room, imagine yourself at the testing center, and answer questions as quickly and accurately as possible.

Keep repeating timed and closed-book tests on a regular basis until you run out of practice tests or it's time for the actual test. Your mind will be ready for the schedule and stress of test day, and you'll be able to focus on recalling the material you've learned.

5

Secret Key #4 – Pace Yourself

Once you're fully prepared for the material on the test, your biggest challenge on test day will be managing your time. Just knowing that the clock is ticking can make you panic even if you have plenty of time left. Work on pacing yourself so you can build confidence against the time constraints of the exam. Pacing is a difficult skill to master, especially in a high-pressure environment, so **practice is vital**.

Set time expectations for your pace based on how much time is available. For example, if a section has 60 questions and the time limit is 30 minutes, you know you have to average 30 seconds or less per question in order to answer them all. Although 30 seconds is the hard limit, set 25 seconds per question as your goal, so you reserve extra time to spend on harder questions. When you budget extra time for the harder questions, you no longer have any reason to stress when those questions take longer to answer.

Don't let this time expectation distract you from working through the test at a calm, steady pace, but keep it in mind so you don't spend too much time on any one question. Recognize that taking extra time on one question you don't understand may keep you from answering two that you do understand later in the test. If your time limit for a question is up and you're still not sure of the answer, mark it and move on, and come back to it later if the time and the test format allow. If the testing format doesn't allow you to return to earlier questions, just make an educated guess; then put it out of your mind and move on.

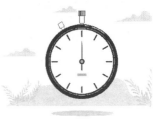

On the easier questions, be careful not to rush. It may seem wise to hurry through them so you have more time for the challenging ones, but it's not worth missing one if you know the concept and just didn't take the time to read the question fully. Work efficiently but make sure you understand the question and have looked at all of the answer choices, since more than one may seem right at first.

Even if you're paying attention to the time, you may find yourself a little behind at some point. You should speed up to get back on track, but do so wisely. Don't panic; just take a few seconds less on each question until you're caught up. Don't guess without thinking, but do look through the answer choices and eliminate any you know are wrong. If you can get down to two choices, it is often worthwhile to guess from those. Once you've chosen an answer, move on and don't dwell on any that you skipped or had to hurry through. If a question was taking too long, chances are it was one of the harder ones, so you weren't as likely to get it right anyway.

On the other hand, if you find yourself getting ahead of schedule, it may be beneficial to slow down a little. The more quickly you work, the more likely you are to make a careless mistake that will affect your score. You've budgeted time for each question, so don't be afraid to spend that time. Practice an efficient but careful pace to get the most out of the time you have.

Secret Key #5 – Have a Plan for Guessing

When you're taking the test, you may find yourself stuck on a question. Some of the answer choices seem better than others, but you don't see the one answer choice that is obviously correct. What do you do?

The scenario described above is very common, yet most test takers have not effectively prepared for it. Developing and practicing a plan for guessing may be one of the single most effective uses of your time as you get ready for the exam.

In developing your plan for guessing, there are three questions to address:

- When should you start the guessing process?
- How should you narrow down the choices?
- Which answer should you choose?

When to Start the Guessing Process

Unless your plan for guessing is to select C every time (which, despite its merits, is not what we recommend), you need to leave yourself enough time to apply your answer elimination strategies. Since you have a limited amount of time for each question, that means that if you're going to give yourself the best shot at guessing correctly, you have to decide quickly whether or not you will guess.

Of course, the best-case scenario is that you don't have to guess at all, so first, see if you can answer the question based on your knowledge of the subject and basic reasoning skills. Focus on the key words in the question and try to jog your memory of related topics. Give yourself a chance to bring the knowledge to mind, but once you realize that you don't have (or you can't access) the knowledge you need to answer the question, it's time to start the guessing process.

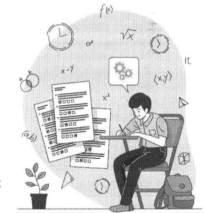

It's almost always better to start the guessing process too early than too late. It only takes a few seconds to remember something and answer the question from knowledge. Carefully eliminating wrong answer choices takes longer. Plus, going through the process of eliminating answer choices can actually help jog your memory.

Summary: Start the guessing process as soon as you decide that you can't answer the question based on your knowledge.

7

How to Narrow Down the Choices

The next chapter in this book (**Test-Taking Strategies**) includes a wide range of strategies for how to approach questions and how to look for answer choices to eliminate. You will definitely want to read those carefully, practice them, and figure out which ones work best for you. Here though, we're going to address a mindset rather than a particular strategy.

Your odds of guessing an answer correctly depend on how many options you are choosing from.

Number of options left	5	4	3	2	1
Odds of guessing correctly	20%	25%	33%	50%	100%

You can see from this chart just how valuable it is to be able to eliminate incorrect answers and make an educated guess, but there are two things that many test takers do that cause them to miss out on the benefits of guessing:

- Accidentally eliminating the correct answer
- Selecting an answer based on an impression

We'll look at the first one here, and the second one in the next section.

To avoid accidentally eliminating the correct answer, we recommend a thought exercise called **the $5 challenge**. In this challenge, you only eliminate an answer choice from contention if you are willing to bet $5 on it being wrong. Why $5? Five dollars is a small but not insignificant amount of money. It's an amount you could afford to lose but wouldn't want to throw away. And while losing

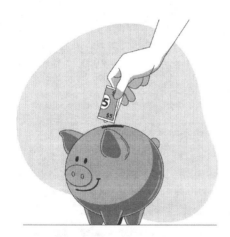

$5 once might not hurt too much, doing it twenty times will set you back $100. In the same way, each small decision you make—eliminating a choice here, guessing on a question there—won't by itself impact your score very much, but when you put them all together, they can make a big difference. By holding each answer choice elimination decision to a higher standard, you can reduce the risk of accidentally eliminating the correct answer.

The $5 challenge can also be applied in a positive sense: If you are willing to bet $5 that an answer choice *is* correct, go ahead and mark it as correct.

Summary: Only eliminate an answer choice if you are willing to bet $5 that it is wrong.

8

Which Answer to Choose

You're taking the test. You've run into a hard question and decided you'll have to guess. You've eliminated all the answer choices you're willing to bet $5 on. Now you have to pick an answer. Why do we even need to talk about this? Why can't you just pick whichever one you feel like when the time comes?

The answer to these questions is that if you don't come into the test with a plan, you'll rely on your impression to select an answer choice, and if you do that, you risk falling into a trap. The test writers know that everyone who takes their test will be guessing on some of the questions, so they intentionally write wrong answer choices to seem plausible. You still have to pick an answer though, and if the wrong answer choices are designed to look right, how can you ever be sure that you're not falling for their trap? The best solution we've found to this dilemma is to take the decision out of your hands entirely. Here is the process we recommend:

Once you've eliminated any choices that you are confident (willing to bet $5) are wrong, select the first remaining choice as your answer.

Whether you choose to select the first remaining choice, the second, or the last, the important thing is that you use some preselected standard. Using this approach guarantees that you will not be enticed into selecting an answer choice that looks right, because you are not basing your decision on how the answer choices look.

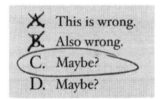

This is not meant to make you question your knowledge. Instead, it is to help you recognize the difference between your knowledge and your impressions. There's a huge difference between thinking an answer is right because of what you know, and thinking an answer is right because it looks or sounds like it should be right.

Summary: To ensure that your selection is appropriately random, make a predetermined selection from among all answer choices you have not eliminated.

Test-Taking Strategies

This section contains a list of test-taking strategies that you may find helpful as you work through the test. By taking what you know and applying logical thought, you can maximize your chances of answering any question correctly!

It is very important to realize that every question is different and every person is different: no single strategy will work on every question, and no single strategy will work for every person. That's why we've included all of them here, so you can try them out and determine which ones work best for different types of questions and which ones work best for you.

Question Strategies

☑ READ CAREFULLY

Read the question and the answer choices carefully. Don't miss the question because you misread the terms. You have plenty of time to read each question thoroughly and make sure you understand what is being asked. Yet a happy medium must be attained, so don't waste too much time. You must read carefully and efficiently.

☑ CONTEXTUAL CLUES

Look for contextual clues. If the question includes a word you are not familiar with, look at the immediate context for some indication of what the word might mean. Contextual clues can often give you all the information you need to decipher the meaning of an unfamiliar word. Even if you can't determine the meaning, you may be able to narrow down the possibilities enough to make a solid guess at the answer to the question.

☑ PREFIXES

If you're having trouble with a word in the question or answer choices, try dissecting it. Take advantage of every clue that the word might include. Prefixes and suffixes can be a huge help. Usually, they allow you to determine a basic meaning. *Pre-* means before, *post-* means after, *pro-* is positive, *de-* is negative. From prefixes and suffixes, you can get an idea of the general meaning of the word and try to put it into context.

☑ HEDGE WORDS

Watch out for critical hedge words, such as *likely, may, can, sometimes, often, almost, mostly, usually, generally, rarely,* and *sometimes.* Question writers insert these hedge phrases to cover every possibility. Often an answer choice will be wrong simply because it leaves no room for exception. Be on guard for answer choices that have definitive words such as *exactly* and *always.*

☑ SWITCHBACK WORDS

Stay alert for *switchbacks.* These are the words and phrases frequently used to alert you to shifts in thought. The most common switchback words are *but, although,* and *however.* Others include *nevertheless, on the other hand, even though, while, in spite of, despite,* and *regardless of.* Switchback words are important to catch because they can change the direction of the question or an answer choice.

⊘ Face Value

When in doubt, use common sense. Accept the situation in the problem at face value. Don't read too much into it. These problems will not require you to make wild assumptions. If you have to go beyond creativity and warp time or space in order to have an answer choice fit the question, then you should move on and consider the other answer choices. These are normal problems rooted in reality. The applicable relationship or explanation may not be readily apparent, but it is there for you to figure out. Use your common sense to interpret anything that isn't clear.

Answer Choice Strategies

⊘ Answer Selection

The most thorough way to pick an answer choice is to identify and eliminate wrong answers until only one is left, then confirm it is the correct answer. Sometimes an answer choice may immediately seem right, but be careful. The test writers will usually put more than one reasonable answer choice on each question, so take a second to read all of them and make sure that the other choices are not equally obvious. As long as you have time left, it is better to read every answer choice than to pick the first one that looks right without checking the others.

⊘ Answer Choice Families

An answer choice family consists of two (in rare cases, three) answer choices that are very similar in construction and cannot all be true at the same time. If you see two answer choices that are direct opposites or parallels, one of them is usually the correct answer. For instance, if one answer choice says that quantity x increases and another either says that quantity x decreases (opposite) or says that quantity y increases (parallel), then those answer choices would fall into the same family. An answer choice that doesn't match the construction of the answer choice family is more likely to be incorrect. Most questions will not have answer choice families, but when they do appear, you should be prepared to recognize them.

⊘ Eliminate Answers

Eliminate answer choices as soon as you realize they are wrong, but make sure you consider all possibilities. If you are eliminating answer choices and realize that the last one you are left with is also wrong, don't panic. Start over and consider each choice again. There may be something you missed the first time that you will realize on the second pass.

⊘ Avoid Fact Traps

Don't be distracted by an answer choice that is factually true but doesn't answer the question. You are looking for the choice that answers the question. Stay focused on what the question is asking for so you don't accidentally pick an answer that is true but incorrect. Always go back to the question and make sure the answer choice you've selected actually answers the question and is not merely a true statement.

⊘ Extreme Statements

In general, you should avoid answers that put forth extreme actions as standard practice or proclaim controversial ideas as established fact. An answer choice that states the "process should be used in certain situations, if…" is much more likely to be correct than one that states the "process should be discontinued completely." The first is a calm rational statement and doesn't even make a definitive, uncompromising stance, using a hedge word *if* to provide wiggle room, whereas the second choice is far more extreme.

11

⏱ BENCHMARK

As you read through the answer choices and you come across one that seems to answer the question well, mentally select that answer choice. This is not your final answer, but it's the one that will help you evaluate the other answer choices. The one that you selected is your benchmark or standard for judging each of the other answer choices. Every other answer choice must be compared to your benchmark. That choice is correct until proven otherwise by another answer choice beating it. If you find a better answer, then that one becomes your new benchmark. Once you've decided that no other choice answers the question as well as your benchmark, you have your final answer.

⏱ PREDICT THE ANSWER

Before you even start looking at the answer choices, it is often best to try to predict the answer. When you come up with the answer on your own, it is easier to avoid distractions and traps because you will know exactly what to look for. The right answer choice is unlikely to be word-for-word what you came up with, but it should be a close match. Even if you are confident that you have the right answer, you should still take the time to read each option before moving on.

General Strategies

⏱ TOUGH QUESTIONS

If you are stumped on a problem or it appears too hard or too difficult, don't waste time. Move on! Remember though, if you can quickly check for obviously incorrect answer choices, your chances of guessing correctly are greatly improved. Before you completely give up, at least try to knock out a couple of possible answers. Eliminate what you can and then guess at the remaining answer choices before moving on.

⏱ CHECK YOUR WORK

Since you will probably not know every term listed and the answer to every question, it is important that you get credit for the ones that you do know. Don't miss any questions through careless mistakes. If at all possible, try to take a second to look back over your answer selection and make sure you've selected the correct answer choice and haven't made a costly careless mistake (such as marking an answer choice that you didn't mean to mark). This quick double check should more than pay for itself in caught mistakes for the time it costs.

⏱ PACE YOURSELF

It's easy to be overwhelmed when you're looking at a page full of questions; your mind is confused and full of random thoughts, and the clock is ticking down faster than you would like. Calm down and maintain the pace that you have set for yourself. Especially as you get down to the last few minutes of the test, don't let the small numbers on the clock make you panic. As long as you are on track by monitoring your pace, you are guaranteed to have time for each question.

⏱ DON'T RUSH

It is very easy to make errors when you are in a hurry. Maintaining a fast pace in answering questions is pointless if it makes you miss questions that you would have gotten right otherwise. Test writers like to include distracting information and wrong answers that seem right. Taking a little extra time to avoid careless mistakes can make all the difference in your test score. Find a pace that allows you to be confident in the answers that you select.

12

⊘ Keep Moving

Panicking will not help you pass the test, so do your best to stay calm and keep moving. Taking deep breaths and going through the answer elimination steps you practiced can help to break through a stress barrier and keep your pace.

Final Notes

The combination of a solid foundation of content knowledge and the confidence that comes from practicing your plan for applying that knowledge is the key to maximizing your performance on test day. As your foundation of content knowledge is built up and strengthened, you'll find that the strategies included in this chapter become more and more effective in helping you quickly sift through the distractions and traps of the test to isolate the correct answer.

Now that you're preparing to move forward into the test content chapters of this book, be sure to keep your goal in mind. As you read, think about how you will be able to apply this information on the test. If you've already seen sample questions for the test and you have an idea of the question format and style, try to come up with questions of your own that you can answer based on what you're reading. This will give you valuable practice applying your knowledge in the same ways you can expect to on test day.

Good luck and good studying!

Cancer Continuum

Biology of Cancer

IMMUNOLOGY

Immunology is the field of medicine that examines the body's ability to fight off infection. The body has a complicated system of cells and certain substances that react when an unknown agent attempts to cause an infectious process within the body. When a cell is altered to form a cancer cell, the body usually recognizes it as abnormal and attacks it. This prevents its replication and the development of more cancer cells. If immune cells are not functioning properly, the cancer cell could go on to reproduce more cells to eventually form a tumor that can potentially invade the surrounding tissues. Immunology also focuses on treatment research and ways in which the immune system can function more effectively in preventing cancer cell formation.

LYMPH ORGANS

Primary lymph organs are responsible for the development of lymphocytes. They also form the receptors to which cancer cells will bind. Primary lymph organs include bone marrow, where B-cells are formed, and the thymus within the mediastinum, where T-cells are developed. The thymus is very active in young people, but becomes inactive later on in adulthood.

Secondary lymph organs are the locations at which cancer cells frequently attempt to take over normal tissues. These include the tonsils, the spleen, organs that can develop cancer, lymph nodes, and bone marrow. The tonsils and organs are able to defend themselves against cancer using lymphatics within the mucosal lining of the organ. The spleen acts as a filter of blood and attempts to destroy abnormal cells as they pass through the organ. Bone marrow is the only lymphatic substance that functions as both primary and secondary lymph tissue.

Lymphocytes are necessary for the body's immune system to function. They are divided into B cells and T cells. B cells are formed in the bone marrow. When a foreign object enters the body, the B cells begin to duplicate and produce immunoglobulins to help function in immunity. T cells mature within the thymus gland and function to produce substances that assist the immune system, help B cells with an immune response, and destroy foreign cells that are present.

Phagocytes are responsible for enclosing foreign substances and destroying them. There are mononuclear phagocytes, polymorphonuclear granulocytes, and eosinophils that aid in this function. **Polymorphonuclear granulocytes** are the most prevalent type of white blood cells and comprise over 50% of the total number of white blood cells. **Basophils** are responsible for traveling to areas where there is tissue injury and causing the release of substances that stimulate an allergic reaction.

DENDRITIC CELLS

Dendritic cells are formed from lymph tissue but most of them come from mononuclear phagocyte cells. They are responsible for activating T cells in fighting foreign cells. It is thought that they are most valuable in immunity against viruses and tumors. When a foreign cell is present in the body, **dendritic cells** take the antigen proteins from the foreign cell and travel through the lymph vessels to deliver the information to the T cells. This stimulates the T cells to formulate an immune response against the foreign cell.

If dendritic cells are not functioning correctly, the T cells cannot receive the antigen protein information from the foreign cell in a timely manner, which can result in a delay in the immune system triggering a response against them. This can result in the development of an infection or the possibility of cancer cells developing and reproducing to form a tumor.

NULL CELLS

Null cells are derived from lymph tissue, but they do not function to activate T cells or B cells. Once they are fully formed, null cells possess an affinity for working with macrophages and neutrophils to trigger an immune response. The two **types of null cells** are natural killer cells and lymphokine-activated cells:

- **Natural killer cells** hold material that functions as enzymes to destroy foreign cells. When the immune response is triggered, natural killer cells function even more efficiently to kill the cells. They have an affinity for virus cells and some tumor cells.
- **Lymphokine-activated cells** are formed outside of the circulatory system by combining lymphocytes with interleukin-2 and then replacing the cells in the patient's body. This creates cells that are much more effective in destroying foreign cells. They do not trigger the activation of other substances within the immune system and must be directly in contact with the foreign cell in order to be effective.

MAST CELLS

Mast cells are **granulocytes**. They have many factors that stimulate the immune system to cause an inflammatory reaction with the tissues where foreign cells or damage has occurred. Mast cells usually reside near blood vessels and can also be found throughout the body within tissues. They appear very similar to basophils and are often mistaken for basophils under the microscope.

The mast cells located within organs are called mucosal mast cells because they are located within the mucosa of the organ. Mast cells that reside near the blood vessels are called connective tissue mast cells.

COMPLEMENT SYSTEM

The complement system is made up of proteins that function in immunity. When a foreign object enters the body, antibodies will attach to it if it is recognizable to them. This activates the complement proteins to travel through the vascular system to the tissue affected. The foreign object, or antigen, is altered when the antibody attaches to it and undergoes changes that allow the complement protein to attach to it as well.

The complement protein causes several activities to occur once it attaches to the antigen. This is often referred to as the **complement cascade**. First, neutrophils and macrophages are activated and they begin to travel to the antigen-antibody article. Other substances are released to cause damage to the cell membrane of the antigen. Enzymes are released to begin breaking down the antigen. The complement system also causes activation of basophils and mast cells, which will stimulate the inflammatory process to further stimulate the immune system into attacking the antigen.

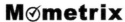

CYTOKINES

Cytokines refer to a group of cells that function to promote maturity of white blood cells and other substances responsible for immunity. They can also trigger other cells within the immune system to function and work with the immune system when necessary.

- **Interferons** are activated in response to viral invasions within the body. They are released early on after exposure to viral agents.
- **Interleukins** are created by T cells, though they are also found within certain tissues.
- **Hematopoietic growth factors**, or colony-stimulating factors, work in organizing and leading cell reproduction. They also trigger the process that distinguishes stem cells from white blood cells.
- **Tumor necrosis factors** are activated in response to inflammation and actions that lead to cell death.
- **Chemokines** are produced by white blood cells and work to direct white blood cells through the body in response to an antigen's presence.

DNA

DNA is the acronym for **deoxyribonucleic acid**. It is the genetic material of life. DNA is found in the nucleus of a cell, which is the spherical structure found in the central region of the cell. Chains of nucleotides create all nucleic acids, with each nucleotide composed of **three essential components**:

- A nitrogen base (pyrimidine or purine)
- A 5-carbon sugar (deoxyribose or ribose)
- A phosphate group

The famous DNA two-strand double helix is formed when four different nucleic acid bases bond loosely to their counterparts. The **purine adenine (A)** binds to the **pyrimidine thymine (T),** and the **purine guanine (G)** binds to the **pyrimidine cytosine (C)**. The resultant double helix makes up a chromosome, of which there are 46 (or 23 pairs) in human cells. There are functional sections within strands of DNA called **genes**. Information contained within the DNA of an individual is inherited, but can also be modified by mutation. The entire array of DNA information is referred to as the **genome**.

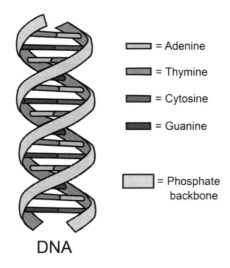

= Adenine

= Thymine

= Cytosine

= Guanine

= Phosphate backbone

DNA

In the human being, the base pairings of DNA are **transcribed** (using a polymerase enzyme) into messenger RNA (mRNA), which can travel out of the nucleus into the cytoplasm or extra-nuclear portion of the cell. The polymerase enzyme temporarily unwinds the DNA strands, and the single strand of DNA acts as a template to form the mRNA transcription from ribonucleic acid (RNA). Structures within the cytoplasm, called ribosomes, **translate** the base pairs in groups of 3 into a code for amino acids, the building blocks of proteins. All living cells, as well as viruses, use proteins as structural and functional components. There are also some sections of the DNA that serve regulatory rather than protein-synthesizing functions.

Pathophysiology of Cancer

FORMATION OF CANCER CELLS

Cancer is a potentially life-threatening disease that occurs due to irregular cell growth and reproduction. These cells can develop into a tumor that can occupy an area where normal body cells are usually found. Cancer cells also have the ability to **metastasize**, or extend, into other areas of the body.

Cells within the body are constantly being replaced by normal cells. During this process, an abnormality in a cell's DNA can occur, which causes it to become a **malignant** cancer cell. The body's immune system will usually attack and destroy this cell, but sometimes there can be a failure of the immune system to do this or the immune system is not able to destroy the cell. When this happens, the cancer cell can continue to reproduce itself until a tumor is formed. Some cancers can even attack normal, healthy cells within the body and alter their DNA so they will begin to reproduce as cancer cells.

> **Review Video: DNA vs. RNA**
> Visit mometrix.com/academy and enter code: 184871

DNA DAMAGE REPAIR AND RESPONSE GENES IN THE MALIGNANT PROCESS

The **malignant process** is controlled by **three types of genes**:

- **Oncogenes**, which are genes that have the potential to convert a normal cell to a cancerous one
- **Tumor suppressor genes**, which are genes that inhibit unrestricted cell division in normal cells but can be inactivated by mutation in cancerous cells
- **DNA damage repair and response genes**

The latter are important because genetic mutations are often inherited in the germ-line. Thus, they can predispose individuals to various types of cancer from birth onward. Pathways to repair human DNA are under the control of a number of genes and involve things like repair of excision errors of nucleotides and bases, or revising mismatches or breaks in the DNA. Mechanisms to repair these DNA problems typically break down in neoplastic cells at various points.

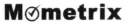

ONCOGENES

Oncogenes are present within the body's cells and play a role in the development of cancer. They are altered portions of the cells' DNA that function to promote the reproduction of cancer cells. The body does have ways of preventing oncogenes from reproducing cancer cells:

- **Proto-oncogenes** make up a portion of the DNA within cells. They are responsible for the replacement of normal cells and also play a role in fixing cells that have been damaged. If proto-oncogenes are altered by cancer cells, they can no longer perform their job of replacing and mending normal cells. These functions will no longer be performed, allowing cancer cells to attack the normal cells in order to produce more cancer cells.
- **Tumor suppression genes** are responsible for halting the replication of cells. They can also function to stop the reproduction of cancer cells. If tumor suppressor genes are altered or damaged, cancer cells will be able to reproduce without any interference.

CELLULAR RESPONSES AFTER DNA DAMAGE

The cellular response pathways after DNA damage are complex. The damage can be endogenous (i.e., internally-derived), such as with spontaneous base changes or replication mistakes. On the other hand, exogenous environmental factors like ultraviolet or ionizing radiation, certain chemicals, or cytotoxic agents can also be introduced to cause DNA changes. The possible outcomes include cell survival, cell death through apoptosis, or malignant transformation via mutation. All of these types of damage initially produce some sort of DNA injury. **Signaling and DNA repair pathways** are subsequently activated, although the signals can differ and thus variously influence the outcome. There is evidence that genes involved with DNA repair can be transcriptionally induced. If DNA damage continues, cellular responses play a role in the eventual outcome. When repair processes are working, they are upregulated and the cell can survive. If the repair processes are insufficient, the cell either dies via apoptosis, or the mutation can initiate malignant transformation.

NUCLEOTIDE EXCISION REPAIR

Nucleotide excision repair (NER) of DNA is a process used to fix many types of lesions that distort the helical formation of double-stranded DNA. The double-stranded configuration aids and promotes this type of repair. There are five steps involved:

1. First, the lesion is recognized.
2. Then factors are recruited to the area to cut away the damaged portion of the strand of DNA.
3. Subsequently, that portion of DNA is excised and removed.
4. Since there is a complementary strand of DNA in the double-helix, that residual strand is used as a template to make a new normal segment of DNA.
5. Lastly, a ligase joins the repaired section to the rest of the DNA strand. This process is also known as **global genomic repair**.

Mutations in genes that regulate nucleotide excision repair have been linked to the inherited propensity towards certain cancers. The most common syndrome associated with defects in nucleotide excision repair is xeroderma pigmentosum (XP), which is characterized by sun sensitivity, pigmentation abnormalities, and predilection to skin cancer development.

BASE EXCISION REPAIR

Metabolic events in the cytoplasm of a cell can oxidize or alkylate DNA and change its base composition. In order for **base excision repair (BER)** to occur, the base damage needs to be identified by a lesion-specific glycosylase, which cuts the base away from its attached sugar. Excision of the DNA area is initiated by either an endonuclease or lyase followed by phosphodiesterase. The area is then repaired by using a DNA polymerase to replicate the original base pairs using the other strand of the DNA as a template. A ligase is then used to join the DNA strand. Malignancies found to be associated with defects in base excision repair include colorectal adenomas, colon cancer, and possibly some lung and breast cancers.

MISMATCH REPAIR

Mismatch repair (MMR) can be required after DNA replication errors, base changes, or other conformational issues arise. These changes result in a mismatch of nucleotides. The steps involved in MMR are fairly similar to other types of repairs:

1. Recognition
2. Conscription of other molecules associated with repair
3. Excision of the mismatched area
4. Replication of a normal DNA sequence and ligation of the repair segment to the residual DNA strand

The most common MMR-associated defect is hereditary nonpolyposis colon cancer. The variant genes predisposing this condition are autosomally dominant, and their presence greatly increases the probability of acquiring this type of malignancy.

DOUBLE-STRAND BREAK REPAIR

Double-strand breaks (DSBs) usually occur in DNA after exposure to certain chemicals or x-rays. They can also be caused by prior single-strand repair errors. There are actually two ways in which DSB repair can occur.

- The first method, known as **non-homologous end-joining**, is quick but has a high incidence of mistakes. Here the two broken ends are simply joined together by recruitment of DNA-dependent protein kinases, other proteins, and ligases through a heterodimer known as Ku70/80.
- The other method, **homologous recombination**, results in far fewer errors. The basic mechanism in this case is the resectioning of some of the single strands through the use of various proteins (mainly RAD and BRCA designations) and nucleases and then the use of a sister molecule as a template.

If double-strand breaks are not properly repaired, dire consequences to the organism can result. In humans, the most common DSB-associated defect is development of the immunodeficiency disease ataxia telangiectasia in which individuals become very susceptible to radiation and prone to various cancers.

CATEGORIES OF CARCINOGENESIS

Carcinogenesis is defined as the process by which normal genes are damaged so that the cells lose control mechanisms and thereby proliferate out of control. Categories include:

- **Familial carcinogenesis** is based on cancer-suppressor genes that are present normally but cause cancer by their absence when changed. Breast cancer is a common example of this.
- **Viral carcinogenesis** in humans has been identified only in a small number of instances (e.g., hepatitis B virus, human T-cell leukemia-lymphoma virus, human papillomaviruses, and Epstein-Barr virus).

- The **bacterial carcinogenesis** by helicobacter pylori is associated with mucosa-associated lymphoid tissue lymphoma.
- **Chemical carcinogenesis** is induced by chemical or toxin exposure (e.g., lung cancer from the smoking of tobacco).
- When secondary smoke causes lung cancer, this is an example of **environmental carcinogenesis**.
- An example of **physical carcinogenesis** is squamous cell cancer caused by exposure to ultraviolet radiation of the sun.

CHARACTERISTICS OF CANCER CELLS

Cancer cells have unique characteristics that make them difficult to kill and prone to multiply:

- **Pleomorphism** means that the cells are of different dimensions and forms.
- **Polymorphism** is the ability of the cell's nucleus to expand and change its form.
- **Hyperchromatism** refers to chromatin within the cell's nucleus that is seen clearly when staining is done for studies.
- **Translocations** are changes in the chromosomes in which genetic information is swapped.
- **Deletions** occur when portions of a chromosome's genetic information are obliterated.
- **Amplification** refers to multiple reproductions of a section of DNA.
- **Aneuploidy** refers to an atypical quantity of chromosomes.

CLASSIFICATIONS OF CANCER GENES

Genes involved with cancer development are classified by functionality into three groups:

- **Gatekeepers**: These genes primarily monitor cell growth (including a number of functions, such as motility, gene repair, adhesion, and cell death) and angiogenesis.
- **Caretakers**: These genes mainly control the stability of the genome and target many of the receptors that are involved in intracellular signaling.
- **Landscapers**: These genes (which are often identified in inborn errors of metabolism and other such hereditary syndromes) produce substances that affect the interaction between the tumor and host microenvironment.

STAGES OF THE DEVELOPMENT OF CANCER

The development of cancer follows stages:

1. **Initiation** is the action of a cancer-causing substance entering the body. Examples include cigarette smoke, radiation exposure, etc. This substance can alter the DNA within the body's cells. The body may respond by fixing the damage and halting the process of cancer cells forming, or the body may not be able to repair the damage that is done. The DNA can go on with these changes without cancer cells being produced, or the DNA can be changed and go on to replicate cancer cells.
2. **Promotion** is the process in which the body is repeatedly exposed to the cancer-causing substance. This repeats the process mentioned above and increases the likelihood of cancer cells being reproduced.
3. **Progression** occurs when the malignant cancer cells begin to outnumber the normal, healthy cells because of continued replication within the body. At this point, the body is no longer able to attempt to repair the damage done to DNA by the cancer-causing agents and the normal cells continue to replicate as cancer cells.

GROWTH CHARACTERISTICS OF CANCER CELLS

Just like normal cells, cancer cells are constantly changing, dying, and reproducing. Different types of tumors **grow** at different rates. This is measured in a percentage of cells that are actively being reproduced at any given time, which is called the **growth fraction**. Tumor growth can also be measured in the amount of time it takes for tumor cells to double in quantity. This is called the **tumor volume doubling time**. Tumors require proper nutrition in order to thrive and continue to grow. To receive the necessary nutrients, there must be blood supply to the tumor. This blood supply is produced through angiogenesis. If the blood supply is not available to the tumor, the tumor cells will die. **Gompertzian growth** is a term that refers to a generality that is made regarding tumor growth. It is thought that tumors grow rapidly early on, but then growth slows down as the tumor enlarges. This most likely occurs due to a lack of the nutrients necessary to thrive.

PROCESSES OF GROWTH, MUTATION, AND MULTIPLICATION

Cancer cells grow, mutate, and multiply in a variety of ways:

- **Hyperplasia** is the process in which the quantity of cells within a certain tissue multiplies. This occurs in healthy tissue and in cancerous tissue.
- **Metaplasia** is when one type of cell is interchanged with another within a specific tissue. This occurs in response to chronic damage inflicted on a certain type of cell.
- **Dysplasia** is a change in normal cells. This can involve a change in any of the cell's characteristics.
- **Anaplasia** refers to the manner in which some cancer stem cells do not differentiate as they multiply. The differentiation of cells is what allows them to function like normal tissue. Anaplastic tumor cells are both visibly and functionally different than the surrounding tissue due to their inability to differentiate, causing them to remain in a stem cell state as they multiply.

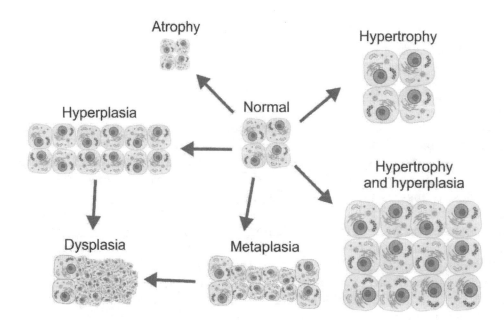

22

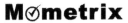

TUMOR PROGRESSION

Tumor development can follow the below progression:

- **Invasion** is the process in which cancer cells continue to reproduce and effectively take over an area of the body's normal, healthy tissue.
- **Angiogenesis** is the process in which a tumor causes the body to produce blood vessels that enable the tumor to survive and grow.
- **Metastasis** is the extension of cancer cells to other parts of the body. This occurs when the cancer cells continue to reproduce and spread into other tissues in the area where the original cancer started. It can also occur through the blood or lymph stream by carrying cancer cells to other tissues within the body. Certain cancers have a propensity for metastasizing to specific areas of the body. For example, prostate and breast cancers are more likely to metastasize to the spine.
- **Tumor heterogeneity** is the term used to describe the dissimilarities found between cancer cells within a tumor. The more heterogeneous a tumor is, the more difficult it can be to treat and the more types of treatments may be required to treat it.

MALIGNANT CHANGES IN TUMOR PROGRESSION

The initial step in tumor development is the appearance of either **hyperplasia** (an enlarged area caused by excessive multiplication of cells) or a **benign tumor** called an adenoma.

If angiogenesis (the formation and differentiation of blood vessels) begins to occur and the stromal cells multiply further, a situation called "carcinoma-in-situ" can develop. **Carcinoma-in-situ** refers to malignancy that is still basically confined to one area and to one associated tissue type. There are various therapies available to target and treat or destroy these tissues.

However, if vascularization and uncontrolled cell growth continues unchecked, the malignancy can eventually invade further and even metastasize to new areas. **Metastasis** is the process by which the malignancy spreads to other areas through the blood and lymphatic systems.

PHENOTYPIC APPEARANCE OF INVASIVE MALIGNANCY

Malignant processes become **invasive** in response to recruitment of a number of factors and cell types. The way in which the surrounding microenvironment and the extracellular matrix are modified is of crucial importance for the switch from simple cellular proliferation to aggressive invasiveness and metastases. Typically, new cell types such as fibroblasts, various types of immune cells, and endothelial cells are recruited to the area. Hypoxia or oxygen deprivation in the area (largely due to abnormally rapid cellular growth) stimulates further production of capillary formation, which provides a direct path for tumor cell migration into the blood system. It also helps to more readily bring a number of growth and regulatory factors into the area, such as tumor necrosis factor, fibroblast growth factor, platelet-derived growth factor, transforming growth factor, and interleukins. Cellular basement membranes gradually break down and signals are transmitted between cells, initiating an increasing cascade of invasive behavior.

INTERACTION BETWEEN RECEPTORS FOR CELL ADHESION AND GROWTH FACTORS

On the surface of a cancerous cell, there are various growth factor receptors, **cell-matrix adhesion receptors** (most notably integrins), **G-protein coupled receptors**, and **receptor-operated calcium channels** (ROCC) as well as other receptors. When **growth factor receptors** and integrins (cell-matrix adhesion receptors) are activated by the appropriate extracellular matrix ligand, they can communicate with or "cross-talk" to each other (when in close proximity) and ultimately send survival and invasiveness signals to the nucleus via a kinase called Akt. Similarly, growth factor

23

receptors can also interact with the G-protein coupled receptor, and integrins can cross-talk to the ROCC. The integrin-ROCC interaction can stimulate mitogen-activated protein kinase, which increases motility and invasiveness—a process in which calcium (Ca^{2+}) plays an important role.

INTERACTION BETWEEN SOLUBLE FACTORS AND CELL ADHESION MOLECULES WITH INVASIVENESS OF CANCER CELLS

When cancer cells become invasive, the number of **cell adhesion molecules (cadherins)** appears to increase, even while growth factor receptors also appear to be stimulated. The cadherins comprise an important class of adhesion molecules. They are composed of type-1 transmembrane proteins that induce cell adhesion, and are dependent on calcium ($Ca2+$) ions to function, hence the name cadherin.

- **E-cadherin** is a substance that is expressed on the epithelial cells of the body. It promotes the integrity and cell-division properties of epithelial cells; its loss appears to be important in the switch to invasiveness.
- When tyrosine kinases are activated, another substance called **B-Catenin** is released; B-Catenin can then translocate to the nucleus where it activates genes related to metastasis via interaction with transcription factors and other genes. Thus, normal intracellular signaling is altered, and invasiveness of cancer cells can result.

TUMOR CELL ANGIOGENESIS

Tumor cell angiogenesis refers to the formation of new blood vessels, which can lead to more rapid tumor progression. There are a number of factors in the extracellular space that appear to either stimulate or slow down this angiogenesis. The current belief, supported by various research studies, is that tumor cells themselves work to induce new blood vessel formation. Localized tumors exist in acidic environments that are also deficient in oxygen and carbohydrates—conditions which promote the production of cytokines. In this instance, one of the most important cytokines is **VEGF**, or **vascular endothelial growth factor**. VEGF promotes endothelial cell growth and movement and also augments the ability of other molecules to penetrate into the blood vessel, in turn promoting further angiogenesis. The demand for nutrients, oxygen, and waste removal, coupled with cellular signaling and communication may all combine to induce angiogenesis. Through this process, new blood vessels extend into the stroma of other cell types, such as connective tissue, allowing the tumor cells to then progress into the stroma.

Often a phenotypic change occurs in which the natural p53 tumor suppressor gene is lost, which results in decreased amounts of a factor that normally inhibits angiogenesis called thrombospondin. The degree of vascularization appears to determine whether a neoplasm is benign or malignant; malignant tumors have much greater blood vessel formation, which increases the probability of the spread of tumor cells.

MECHANISMS BY WHICH TUMOR CELLS CAN BECOME INVASIVE

Tumor cells have to break through the surrounding connective tissue or stroma in order to become **invasive**. The basement membrane of the stroma must be penetrated for this to occur. There are basically three methods of penetration. Sometimes this penetration can occur through simple pushing of the tumor mass through stromal sites. Another mechanism is augmented tumor cell motility or movement associated with the loss of cohesive forces between cells. This results primarily from suppressed levels of E-cadherin, and the associated alteration of other factors. Tumor cells also produce enzymes that can break down basement membranes. Invasiveness has also been associated with the loss of receptors, such as integrin, during progression of the disease, ultimately leading to cellular detachment.

DEVELOPMENT OF HETEROGENEOUS POPULATIONS IN METASTASES FROM SINGLE CLONES OF MALIGNANT CELLS

Cancerous tumors and neoplasms can metastasize to varying degrees. In most cases, metastases are derived from a **single clone**. However, metastatic cells often have genetic changes, such as deletions, insertions, areas that have been rearranged, or an unusual number of chromosomes. These genetic abnormalities, together with the microenvironment of the host tissues, appear to decrease the stability of the genome of tumor cells. Thus, the mutation rate in these cells is greatly enhanced. Due to this, heterogeneous populations of cells often develop within cancerous tumors, even though the original source was a single clone. This also makes it more difficult to develop treatment plans for cancer patients, because the tumor cell population can continue to change.

DEVELOPMENT OF METASTASES

The development of metastases is a multi-step process that can be arrested in theory at any point. Generally, the steps are as follows:

1. Some process occurs that transforms normal cells into malignant ones.
2. Angiogenesis or new blood vessel formation then occurs.
3. Some of the tumor cells begin to spread into the surrounding stroma, usually via the lymphatic system or blood vessels.
4. Tumor cells or masses subsequently detach and embolize, or stick to blood components in the circulation.
5. A portion of these cells persist in the circulation.
6. Tumor cells ultimately settle in certain organs by adhering to some portion of the vascular wall of a blood vessel perfusing that area.
7. Extravasation or leakage of the tumor cells into the surrounding tissues next takes place.
8. Finally, new proliferation or rapid multiplication of cells occurs in the new site, and a new cycle of metastasis may begin.

> **Review Video: Cancer Classification and Metastasis**
> Visit mometrix.com/academy and enter code: 878417

METASTASES INTO THE LYMPHATIC SYSTEM VERSUS INTO THE BLOODSTREAM

Tumors can **metastasize** into both the **lymphatic system** and the **bloodstream**. These processes are not necessarily mutually exclusive, and passage between each of these systems can occur. As they become invasive, tumor cells can pass into small lymphatic vessels. A portion of these cells may become trapped in regional lymph nodes (RLNs) causing enlargement of the area. For example, melanoma metastasis seems to be highly correlated with entrapment at RLNs. Other tumor cells may escape the RLNs and thus emerge as metastases elsewhere. If tumor cells get into the bloodstream instead, most will die in the circulation. Thus, the metastatic tumor burden depends on the number of cells that initially penetrated the bloodstream. The site of deposition of the metastatic cells depends on factors influencing their adherence to the cell wall, including aggregation of the tumor cells to each other or in combination with lymphocytes or platelets. Subsequently, extravasation into the surrounding tissues can occur.

PROLIFERATION OF METASTATIC TUMOR CELLS AT SECONDARY SITES

Cancer cells can travel from the site of origin to **secondary sites** and there exist as single cells or metastases. The probability of metastases occurring in particular organs appears to be related to a number of factors. The concentrations of certain hormones and paracrine or autocrine growth factors in the host organ have been highly associated with the proliferation of tumor cells in specific organs. Many of these factors are highly expressed in the liver, for example, including insulin-like

25

growth factor-I, the tumor growth factors, and others. In order to survive and grow in their new microenvironment, the metastatic cells take over some of the mechanisms within the host organ that would normally keep them in a state of equilibrium.

SECONDARY METASTASES

Cancer can metastasize from its original site. Metastases consist of the original tumor's tissues. Thus, breast cancer that metastasizes to the lungs is known as metastatic breast cancer, not lung cancer. **Metastasis of metastases,** also known as **secondary metastases,** can also occur. If new blood vessels are infiltrated by malignant cells at the initial metastatic site, they can reenter the circulation and subsequently produce metastases at other sites by a new cycle. Cancer cells are particularly prone to metastases because they do not adhere well to each other. Thus, they more easily break free and migrate away. Most of the research in this area has been performed in animal models utilizing mice.

APOPTOSIS

Apoptosis is a term meaning programmed cell death. It is a process that occurs in multicellular organisms. Apoptosis can occur in two ways. Apoptosis occurs when various tumor necrosis factors bind to cell-surface "death" receptors and activate caspase and other substances that promote cell death. Apoptosis also occurs when the cellular mitochondria are destroyed and release their contents, including cytochrome c, which eventually activates another caspase that destroys the cell. The latter mechanism is initially triggered by the interaction of a growth factor receptor with a ligand. There is a family of proteins called Bcl-2 that appears to regulate the integrity of mitochondria and contributes to the second method of apoptosis.

TRIGGERING FACTORS IN CANCER CELLS

An oncogene is a gene that has the potential to induce a normal cell to become cancerous. In some cases, oncogenes appear to stimulate cell death by programming the release of apoptotic substances from the mitochondria. The mechanism of this **triggering of apoptosis** has not been pinpointed, but activation of the c-Myc oncogene (a family of genes that are consistently over-expressed in the presence of cancer) appears to play a role. Other factors are also involved. If a cell escapes death, it must still stimulate other processes, such as growth and division, which are also controlled to some extent by oncogenes. Cell death can also be incited by a number of tumor suppressors including p53 (and its stimulants), members of the Bcl-2 family, and another protein, called PTEN, coded on chromosome 10.

FACTORS THAT PREVENT CELL DEATH AND PERMIT CANCER CELLS TO PROLIFERATE

Some members of the Bcl-2 family enhance **survival of cancer cells** instead of their death. These antiapoptotic proteins are highly expressed in certain types of cancers, particularly lymphoma. Another way cancer cells can escape cell death is by activation of NF-kB. If the normal inhibitor of this factor is absent, the NF-kB can translocate to the nucleus unchecked, where it can induce genes that inhibit cell death. There is also another conduit by which cancer cell survival can occur involving phosphotidylinositol-3-kinase (PI3K) and another molecule called serine/threonine kinase Akt. Akt overexpression has been associated with a number of malignancies. This pathway is stimulated by a number of growth factors, and the survival enhancing mechanism may focus on the preservation of the integrity of the mitochondria.

WAYS CELL DEATH CAN BE TURNED OFF WITHOUT MUTATION

It has been demonstrated that the chemical transformation of cellular genetic material can **turn off the mechanisms of apoptosis,** even though no mutation has occurred. These events are termed epigenetic, which means they are not associated with actual changes in the DNA. Epigenetic cell survival mechanisms include methylation and histone deacetylation. Proteins that promote tumor suppressor genes, such as caspase, are often methylated (containing 5-methylcytosine where there should be cytosine at the C5 position on DNA); substances that inhibit this methylation have been investigated as therapeutic regimens. If histones are deactivated, genes triggering cell death can also be turned off, probably by obscuring transcription factors. When methods of apoptosis have been suppressed by epigenetic mechanisms, tumors can be unresponsive to normal chemotherapeutic agents.

CURRENT CANCER THERAPY APPROACHES THAT ATTEMPT TO RESTORE APOPTOTIC ABILITY

The basis for most cancer chemotherapy regimens is the **restoration of apoptosis of the malignant cells**. There are a number of ways to restore apoptosis, such as the reintroduction of genes for wild-type proteins like p53 on adenoviral vectors, exposing the cell to proteins that promote lysis, using small molecules to bring back functionality of p53, and possibly introducing inhibitors of epigenetic methylation or histone deacetylation. Various ways of inhibiting different molecules that allow cell survival are currently being investigated. These include not only the use of suppressors of known cell survival factors, but also genetic approaches involving antisense oligonucleotides that complement and block translation of portions of the DNA. Ligands binding to receptors that result in ultimate cell death, like tumor necrosis factor, can kill cancerous and normal cells nonselectively, in general. But a variant called the TRAIL variant may prove to be of greater and more selective value.

Causes of Cancer

CARCINOGENS AND PROCARCINOGENS

A **carcinogen** is any substance or agent that can potentially cause cancer. The term refers more specifically to an agent or substance that can produce epithelial malignancies or carcinomas. Carcinogenic chemicals usually need to be converted into **procarcinogens**, or more stable and reactive intermediate forms, in order to effectively induce the genetic mutations that can lead to cancer. Carcinogenic agents fall into several categories. Some of the most widespread causes of cancer arise from cultural habits like cigarette smoking and exposure to radiation from the sun. Many other causative agents are occupational hazards, such as exposure to organic chemicals like benzene, coal tars, and ethylene oxide in the workplace. Various prescription drugs have been associated with the development of cancers, including estrogens and immune suppressants. Further, a relationship between exposure to certain infectious agents and a particular cancer type has been found in some cases.

MOST COMMON CAUSES OF CANCER

The most common documented causes of cancer include the following:

1. **Radiation** can cause cancer by altering a cell's DNA. If the body is not able to repair the damages, the cell can reproduce as a cancer cell. Radiation exposure can be accidental or from diagnostic testing. UV light exposure is also a form of radiation and causes skin cancer. Asbestos is considered a form of radiation as well and causes mesothelioma tumors within the lungs.
2. **Chemical carcinogens** can alter a cell's DNA to cause cancer. An example of this is cigarette smoke and exposure to tar within cigarettes.
3. **Viruses** can cause cancer. Viruses that alter a cell's genetic material can stimulate the production of cancer cells.

4. The **immune system** may be unsuccessful in repairing or destroying cells with altered DNA, which can lead to cancer. Certain cancer cells have the ability to alter the immune system so that it cannot recognize the formation of malignant cells within normal tissues.
5. Cancer can also occur because of **inherited factors**. A person can inherit oncogenes responsible for causing certain types of cancer.

CARCINOGENIC CHEMICALS

Chemicals that have been found to be carcinogenic fall into several categories. Most are organic chemicals, although some inorganic metals have **carcinogenic potential** as well. The major types include:

- **Polycyclic aromatic hydrocarbons (PAHs), in particular benzo[a]pyrene (B[a]P)**: Originally identified in coal tar, B[a]P is carcinogenic. It is primarily associated with certain occupations, as well as tobacco exposure, and is linked to many types of cancers.
- **Aromatic amines**: These are organic compounds with distinctive smells. This category includes some dyes, benzidine, and naphthylamine, and most often associated with bladder cancer.
- **Benzene**: Benzene is found in petroleum products and solvents and linked to development of leukemia.
- **Aflatoxins**: Aflatoxins are produced by *Aspergillus* fungal strains. Found in certain contaminated food products, this category is linked to liver cancer (perhaps in association with Hepatitis B virus).
- **Chemicals found in tobacco smoke**: Encompassing at least 30 carcinogenic chemicals, including PAHs, aromatic amines, N-Nitrosamines, inorganic metals and more. This category is typically associated with lung cancer and a variety of other malignancies.

CARCINOGENIC METALS

There are four major inorganic metals that have been classified as carcinogenic. They are all present to some extent in tobacco, and all are linked to lung cancer. The **carcinogenic metals** include the following:

- **Arsenic**: Found in some pesticides, some gold ores, and the copper smelting industry; associated with certain skin cancers
- **Cadmium**: Documented weak association with prostate cancer
- **Chromates**: Carcinogenic potential related to the valency of the chromium involved
- **Nickel**: Associated with nasal and laryngeal cancers

RADIATION EXPOSURE AND CANCER DEVELOPMENT

Exposure to different wavelengths of **radiation** has been linked to the development of various cancers. Exposure to the ultraviolet wavelengths by sunlight is the major cause of skin cancer. The carcinogenic potential of sunlight appears to be restricted to the UV-B portion with wavelengths between 280 and 320 nanometers, because that is the area of overlap with the DNA absorption spectrum. Pigmentation of the skin plays a role in susceptibility to the effects of ultraviolet radiation. Dark-skinned individuals are less prone to the development of basal cell or squamous cell carcinoma and the most dangerous type of skin cancer, melanoma. The primary means of overexposure to ionizing radiation, on the other hand, is through the taking of x-rays or through therapeutic procedures utilizing x-rays. Overexposure to x-rays has been linked to a variety of cancer types. The radioactive decay and production of alpha particles by radon gas in the mining industry has been connected to lung cancer as well.

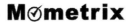

DUSTS AND FIBERS ASSOCIATED WITH CARCINOGENESIS

Certain **dusts and fibers** have been found to be carcinogenic. For example, a number of industries have used asbestos for manufacturing, insulation, or other reasons. Asbestos was an appealing product due to its resilience to decay, molds, and mildew and its heat-resistant properties. However, it also gives off silicate fibers with carcinogenic potential. In a number of studies, asbestos has been linked to lung cancers as well as to growths in the pleura, peritoneum, larynx, and gastrointestinal tract. Therefore, it is rarely used today. Other silica dusts are generated in industries like mining and pottery production, and again, an association with lung cancer has been established. Exposure to wood dusts in occupations like lumberjacking or paper mill works has primarily been linked to nasal adenocarcinoma.

DIETARY SOURCES OF CARCINOGENS AND ANTICARCINOGENS

The process of carcinogenesis is very complex, but studies have shown relationships between **dietary intake** and development of tumors, or the lack thereof. There appears to be an association between fat consumption and development of malignancies that are hormone-dependent, such as endometrial, breast, ovarian, and prostate cancer. The incidence of cancers involving parts of the intestinal tract is increased with high fat consumption as well. The latter includes colon cancer, the incidence of which is also increased in populations who eat a great deal of red meat. Fat consumption and/or the production of substances like PAHs and aromatic amines during cooking may also play specific roles in the carcinogenic process. Calorie restriction in animals generally appears to depress cancer rates, suggesting an association between calories consumed and possible carcinogenesis. There are also components in food, such as certain vitamins, minerals, and *Beta*-carotene, which seem to act as anticarcinogens and lower cancer rates, primarily through their antioxidant effects.

ENVIRONMENTAL CARCINOGENS

There are several ways that scientists have looked for evidence of **exposure to environmental carcinogens**, but here we will focus on the most common two. The first of these approaches has been to develop bioassays that look for the possible carcinogen directly. These bioassays react to the presence of the target carcinogen when coupled with DNA or attached to proteins, either in the tissues themselves or when excreted in the urine. Some bioassays look for metabolites of the carcinogenic agent in the urine. The second approach has been to quantify biological response markers. This tactic involves looking for markers that are associated with human susceptibility to various environmental factors. These types of studies have looked for differences in DNA sequences that are linked to metabolic pathways, or for the inability to repair cellular DNA, as well as other markers.

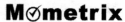

Cancer Epidemiology and Risk Factors

EPIDEMIOLOGIC DATA

Cancer epidemiology involves many statistical quantities. Below is a list of some of the quantities important to cancer epidemiology. Most of these quantities are stated either as a percentage or as a number of cases per 100,000 individuals. Most of these statistics can be found not only as aggregated (all cancers) statistics but also broken out by type of cancer, gender, ethnicity, and other characteristics.

- **Incidence rate** refers to the number of **new** cases that are diagnosed in a given time period, typically a year. It is reported as the number of cases per 100,000 individuals.
- **Prevalence rate** refers to the total number of cases that were **active** during any part of a given time period, typically a year. It is reported as the number of cases per 100,000 individuals. Prevalence rates are always higher than incidence rates for the same time period since prevalence rates count all the same cases that incidence rates do plus all previously diagnosed cases that are still active.
- **Mortality rate** (or **death rate**) refers to the number of people who died from a particular disease during a given time period, typically a year. It is reported as the number of deaths per 100,000 individuals.
- **Case-fatality rate** (CFR) refers to the mortality rate among only those diagnosed with a particular disease. It is reported as a percentage. CFR is a useful metric for evaluating how deadly a particular type of cancer is or comparing among different types of cancer.
- **Survival rate** refers to the likelihood of living at least a given length of time, usually 5 or 10 years, after having been diagnosed with a particular disease. It is reported as a percentage.
- **Absolute risk** refers to the likelihood of being diagnosed with a particular disease in a given time period. This time period can be stated as a set length of time (e.g., within five years), prior to given age (e.g., before the age of 40), or at any point in an individual's entire lifetime. It can be expressed as a percentage or as numerical odds (e.g., 12 out of 100,000). Percentages are typically preferred when the value is at least 0.1%.
- **Relative risk** refers to the likelihood of being diagnosed with a particular disease among those subject to an identified risk factor for the disease. Risk factors may be intrinsic (e.g., age, gender, ethnicity, BMI, other diseases present), behavioral (e.g., smoking, drinking alcohol, sedentary lifestyle), or environmental (e.g., air quality, substance exposure). Relative risk is expressed in the same terms as absolute risk.
- **Attributable risk** refers to difference in likelihood of being diagnosed with a particular disease between those exposed to a risk factor and those not exposed. It essentially expresses how much of a person's risk for a disease is due to a particular risk factor (e.g., how much more likely is someone to develop lung cancer given that they smoke?).

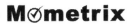

NON-MODIFIABLE RISK FACTORS FOR CANCER

Cancer risks can be divided into modifiable and non-modifiable categories. **Non-modifiable cancer risks** are those that cannot be controlled by changes in human action. Examples include the following:

- **Age**: As individuals advance in age, so does their risk for cancer, with the median age for diagnosis of most cancers being over the age of 60.
- **Gender**: Excluding sex-specific cancers, such as prostate and breast cancer, males have a higher risk of developing and dying from cancer, both in childhood and in adulthood.
- **Cancer history**: Generally, individuals who have had cancer in the past have a higher likelihood of developing a new cancer as compared to those of similar age, race, and sex who have not had cancer previously.

MODIFIABLE RISK FACTORS FOR CANCER

The likelihood of development of cancers can be diminished greatly by the avoidance of a number of **modifiable risk factors**:

- The ultimate preventative measure is **smoking cessation**, because tobacco smoke and associated chemicals are the major carcinogens responsible for lung cancer and many other tumors.
- **Infectious agents** have been recognized as factors in the development of a number of cancers, and screening procedures can identify the presence of these agents and direct therapeutic regimens.
- Many **substances** have been classified as possible carcinogens, and they can be avoided. These types of chemicals range from asbestos and aniline dyes to hormones.
- Certain **dietary changes** have been found to decrease cancer risk, such as ingestion of high-fiber foods or drinking moderate levels of red wine (which contains resveratrol, which is also found in grape skin, for those who do not drink alcohol).

Some other relatively modifiable risk factors include:

- **Geographical location**: According to the CDC, geographic location alone can be a risk factor for cancer. They have identified ten states that have noticeably higher rates of new cancer development: Connecticut, Delaware, Iowa, Kentucky, Louisiana, Maine, Michigan, New Hampshire, New York, and Pennsylvania. Additionally, certain rural locations may emit more toxins if chemical plants are abundant, while certain urban locations may emit toxins from transportation services and high human density.
- **Occupation**: Certain occupations predispose individuals to cancer due to exposure and lifestyle. Sedentary jobs increase the risk for cancer in the same way that obesity does. Shift work puts stresses on the circadian rhythm, which has been linked to increased risk of cancer (among other disease). Other risk factors include professions with heavy sun exposure, exposure to rubber manufacturing, asbestos exposure, and radon or uranium exposure (common to miners working underground).

SMOKING POPULATION TRENDS

Across most racial classifications, the percentage of men who smoke is greater than the proportion of women who smoke. Nevertheless, the quit-rate for women who smoke is lower than the quit-rate for men. Since women are susceptible to some cancers that do not generally affect men, such as cervical cancer, this is an area of concern. According to the CDC, about 14% of individuals in the United States smoke, which has decreased over the last decade. The rate is highest among Native

Americans and fairly similar for Caucasians and African Americans. However, the quit-rate in these two groups is much different. African Americans appear to have more difficulty in adhering to smoking cessation protocols. The prevalence of depression and related disorders is higher among smokers, and these feelings tend to be enhanced during cessation protocols. This may contribute to a lowered incidence of success in these individuals. Success rates also appear to be impacted by the presence of positive support or the lack of negative social factors. Intensive cessation protocols for high-risk groups, such as cancer patients and pregnant women, have produced relatively high quit-rates.

ETHNIC GROUPING AND CANCER

Culture or ethnic factors that influence cancer are many and varied. The most affected ethnic group overall are **African Americans**, who have the highest rate of cancer from all sources; more than any other ethnic group. The group with the lowest rate of cancer overall is **Native Americans.** Prostate cancer incidence is highest in African American males. The **Japanese** have the highest 5-year survival rate from all types of cancer; whereas the Native Americans have the lowest 5-year survival rate. One factor common to all groups and influencing all groups is the **lower socio-economic class**. This class has the highest incidence of cancer regardless of the ethnic group.

EFFECTS OF POVERTY ON PATIENTS WITH CANCER

Poverty is exhibited more in **minorities** than others in this country and these individuals have a poorer prognosis when diagnosed with cancer than those who are not minorities. The most obvious reason may be because of a **lack of medical resources**. Health insurance may not be available for this group of people because they cannot afford it, or they may have low-paying jobs that do not offer insurance benefits. Lack of education and possible distrust for the medical system can also lead to an unclear understanding of their disease and poor compliance with treatment.

Patients who are poverty-stricken may not be able to participate in **regular screening practices** to help with cancer prevention and early detection. This can be due to a lack of understanding or because of low income or no insurance.

Poor nutritional status and **poor living conditions** can also contribute to a poorer prognosis with cancer in a poverty-stricken patient.

HEALTH DISPARITIES AND CANCER INCIDENCE AND DEATH RATES

The term *health disparities* describes the concept of a disease or class of diseases having a measurably different impact on different subsets of a population, usually applied to distinct ethnic groups. According to the National Cancer Institute's Surveillance, Epidemiology, and End Results (SEER) Program, statistics indicate that cancer health disparities exist across major ethnic groups in the United States. The two major statistics that are published in this regard are cancer incidence rate and cancer death rate. **Cancer incidence rate** is the rate at which patients are newly diagnosed with cancer annually, measured in cases per 100,000 individuals. For example, if a group includes 10 million individuals and 5250 of them are newly diagnosed with cancer in a given year, the cancer incidence rate for that group is 52.5 per 100,000. The **cancer death rate** is the rate at which individuals die as a result of cancer annually, measured in deaths per 100,000 individuals. For example, in that same group, if 2430 individuals die from cancer, the cancer death rate is 24.3 per 100,000 for that year.

According to the most recent available data from the SEER Program (2013-2017), the **cancer incidence rate** was highest for the Caucasian population (451.1 per 100,000) and lowest for the Asian/Pacific Islander population (302.1 per 100,000). The **cancer death rate** for the same period

32

was highest for the African American population (181.7 per 100,000) and lowest for the Asian/Pacific Islander population (98.9 per 100,000). Below are the statistics in full:

Rates per 100,000	Incidence Rate	Death Rate
All U.S.	442.4	158.3
Caucasian	**451.1**	159.0
African American	440.4	**181.7**
Hispanic	348.4	112.3
Asian/Pacific Islander	302.1	98.9
American Indian/Alaska Native	310.1	144.2

Caucasian women have the highest rate of new cancer diagnoses among all women, and African American men have the highest rate of new cancer diagnoses among all men.

COLORECTAL CANCER

Colorectal cancer is the third most commonly diagnosed cancer in both men and women. Among men in 2016, African Americans had the **highest incidence** of colorectal cancer (50 per 100,000), while Asians/Pacific Islanders had the **lowest** (36.3 per 100,000). Meanwhile among women, American Indians/Alaskan Natives and African Americans were tied for the **highest** incidence of colorectal cancer at about 37 per 100,000, while Asians/Pacific Islanders were again the **lowest** in this category (25.4 per 100,000). **Death rates** for colorectal cancer in men largely reflect the incidence rates, with African Americans having the **highest** rate (23 per 100,000), and Asians/Pacific Islanders having the lowest (10.6 per 100,000). Among women, African Americans had the **highest** death rates from colorectal cancer (15.1 per 100,000), while Hispanics and Asians/Pacific Islanders tied for the **lowest** death rates at about 8 per 100,000.

LUNG CANCER

Lung cancer is the second most common cancer diagnosis, but is the most common cause of cancer death. Among men in 2016, African Americans had the **highest** incidence (68.1 per 100,000) and death rate (55.3 per 100,000) for lung cancer with Caucasians second highest in both categories (58.8 and 47.1 per 100,000, respectively). Among women, Caucasians had the **highest** incidence rate (49.6 per 100,000) and death rate (33.2 per 100,000), with African Americans second in both categories (42.1 and 29.8 per 100,000, respectively). Meanwhile, Hispanics of both sexes had the **lowest** incidence and death rates in for lung cancer in 2016.

PROSTATE CANCER

Prostate cancer is the most common cancer diagnosis among men, and third most common cancer diagnosis overall. It is the second leading cause of cancer death in men, second to lung cancer. In 2016, African Americans had the **highest** incidence rate (170.2 per 100,000) and death rate (38.4 per 100,000) among all men. Caucasians were second in prostate cancer incidence, at a rate of 98.9 per 100,000, while American Indians/Alaskan Natives were tied with Caucasians for second in prostate cancer death rate at about 18 per 100,000. Asians/Pacific Islanders had the **lowest** incidence rate (52.9 per 100,000) and death rate (8.5 per 100,000) for prostate cancer.

BREAST CANCER

Breast cancer is the most common cancer diagnosis in women, as well as the most common cancer diagnosis overall. It is the second leading cause of cancer death in women, second to lung cancer. Among women in 2016, Caucasians had the **highest** incidence rate of breast cancer (128.9 per 100,000), with African Americans second (123 per 100,000). American Indians/Alaskan Natives had the **lowest** incidence rate for breast cancer (73.6 per 100,000). African Americans had the

33

highest death rate from breast cancer (27.3 per 100,000), with Caucasians second (19.6 per 100,000). Asians/Pacific Islanders had the **lowest** death rate from breast cancer (10.6 per 100,000).

LUNG CANCER RISK FACTORS

Lung cancer causes more deaths in both men and women in this country than any other type of cancer. Approximately 90% of all people who develop lung cancer are **smokers**. There are known risks for lung cancer with second-hand exposure to smoke, but no exact figures are known for incidence of cancer in this population. It is known that when smokers quit smoking, some repair occurs within the lung tissue. This does not immediately decrease the risk of developing lung cancer, but the risk will begin to decrease at least 5 years after quitting smoking.

Other factors that increase the risk of developing lung cancer include **environmental exposure to carcinogens**, such as asbestos, uranium, and radon.

Overall, lung cancer has a very **poor prognosis**, though this depends on how advanced the disease is at the time of diagnosis and whether metastasis develops. The 5-year survival rate for non-small cell lung cancer is approximately 15%, whereas the survival rate for small cell lung cancers is approximately 5%.

BLADDER CANCER RISK FACTORS

Men are three times more likely to develop bladder cancer than women. The risk is increased in men over the age of 60, and Caucasians are twice as likely to develop bladder cancer as African Americans. The incidence of bladder cancer has slowly increased over time.

- **Smoking cigarettes** has been proven to be the most likely cause in over one-half of all cases of bladder cancers in men. About one-quarter of all bladder cancers in women are linked to cigarette smoking.
- Working with certain **industrial chemicals** also places a person more at risk for developing bladder cancer. The industries that show the highest incidence of bladder cancer include paint manufacturing, textiles, and leathers.
- **Poor dietary habits** and frequently eating fried or fatty foods increase the risk of developing bladder cancer. The fat-soluble vitamins A and E have shown to help prevent the formation of bladder malignancies as well as the mineral zinc.

PROSTATE CANCER RISK FACTORS

The incidence of prostate cancer has gradually decreased, which is most likely due to more screening being performed with prostate specific antigen (PSA) testing. Overall, prostate cancer accounts for 1 in 3 cancers in men. The prognosis for patients with prostate cancer has slowly improved in all groups except for African American males.

- Prostate cancer is more common in **older men**, and it has been found that prostate cancer affects over one-half of men 90-years-old or older.
- Prostate cancer is more likely to occur in **African American men** than Caucasian men.
- There is a proven **genetic link** to prostate cancer, and men whose female relatives had breast cancer may also be at an increased risk for prostate cancer.
- Men who work in the **farming industry** or in the **manufacture of batteries** are more susceptible to prostate cancer than others. This is due to an increased exposure to the element cadmium.

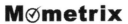

HEAD AND NECK CANCER RISK FACTORS

Most cancers that occur in the head and neck occur in the mouth. The second most common is laryngeal cancer following by oropharyngeal cancer. Men are more likely than women to develop a head or neck cancer and these are more common in people over the age of 50.

- **Smoking** is the number one risk factor that greatly increases the chance of developing head and neck cancer.
- **Alcoholism** greatly increases the risk for mouth cancer and cancer of the pharynx.
- **Chewing tobacco** can greatly increase the risk for oral cancer.
- Cancers that occur on the outside of the mouth are mostly caused by **UV, or sunlight, exposure.**
- **Carcinogenic inhalants**, such as cigarette smoke, asbestos, or wood dust, can greatly increase the risk for cancers of the nasal passages, nasopharynx, or larynx.
- Cancers of the oropharynx are usually caused by **excessive alcohol consumption** or can even result from **poor oral hygiene**.

COLORECTAL CANCER RISK FACTORS

Patients over the age of 50 have a much greater chance of developing colorectal cancer than those who are younger.

- Patients who **do not have access to or do not choose** to have regular screening procedures for colon cancer may develop the disease and not know until symptoms become bothersome. This puts them at risk for having more advanced disease if they do develop colon cancer.
- **Chronic inflammatory diseases** that involve the colon, rectum, and anus can increase the chances for developing colon cancer. These include Crohn's disease, ulcerative colitis, or a history of villous adenoma polyps.
- Patients with **diets high in fat and low in fiber** are more likely to develop colon cancer. Those who work in environments in which they are exposed to air particles from wood or metal manufacturing are also at risk.
- A **family history** of colon cancer or familial polyposis also increases the chance for developing colon cancer.

HUMAN PAPILLOMAVIRUS AND CERVICAL CANCER

Some types of the sexually transmitted disease human papillomavirus (HPV) cause cancer. Approximately 26,000 cases of cancer diagnosed each year are directly attributable to HPV. The CDC recommends an **HPV vaccine** for females 13-26 years of age and for males 13-21 years of age. There are two vaccines available, Gardasil and Cervarix, and both are indicated for the prevention of human papillomavirus-associated diseases including cervical cancer, genital warts, vulvar neoplasia, and vaginal neoplasia. The vaccines are not 100% reliable in the prevention of cervical cancer and does not protect against all causes of gynecological malignancies or sexually transmitted infections. No pretreatment laboratory tests are required. Patient with an allergy to yeast should not receive this vaccine. The drug is administered as an IM injection and given in three separate doses. The vaccine has been proven to be most effective when all three doses have been given before the patient begins sexual activity. Side effects include headache, nausea/vomiting, fainting, fever, and irritation and pain at the injection site.

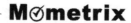

Hereditary Factors in Cancer Development

CANCER GENETICS

There are a variety of tests available to look for **genetic markers**. Information about the genetic makeup of an individual as it relates to cancer is used in several ways. This information is often utilized in patient management, either to aid in diagnosis of different cancers or to evaluate a prognosis for the individual. Knowledge of the presence of genetic markers can also aid in the selection of therapeutic regimens. The other way in which testing for genetic markers can be used is to counsel people regarding their genetic reproductive risk, including the risk for development of cancers in their children, or to assess the probability of the occurrence of cancer in the individuals themselves.

CANCER GENETIC COUNSELING

The first step in cancer genetic counseling should be a frank discussion between the counselor and the patient regarding their preconceptions. Then a complete pedigree of the individual's family needs to be constructed, including documentation of malignancies and other conditions. A medical history and physical examination should be done on the patient with emphasis on any factors that might indicate a propensity toward development of cancer. At that point, the person is usually counseled about cancer risk based on their pedigree, medical history, and physical examination. The counselor develops a plan for further diagnostic and prognostic tests, discusses it with the patient, and institutes the plan if informed consent is obtained from the individual. There are numerous components that should be discussed before obtaining informed consent. Lastly, a strategy for patient follow-up should be established to ensure monitoring where necessary and continued support as needed.

INFORMED CONSENT IN GENETIC TESTING FOR CANCER

Informed consent is a process by which a patient or subject is informed of every substantive aspect of any medical procedure before he or she agrees in writing to have it performed. In the case of genetic testing for cancer, there are certain specific ethical and psychological issues that also need to be covered. The purpose, diagnostic value, and accuracy of the tests need to be explained to the individual, as well as other diagnostic options. Since these are genetic tests, information about risk of transmission to progeny and the possibility of other family members having the gene need to be explained. Ethically, the patient needs to know how confidential the gleaned information will be kept and whether job security or the ability to obtain insurance might be affected by the results. Also, the patient needs to understand that many of these procedures are considered nonessential and thus may not be covered by insurance.

GENETIC COMPONENTS OF BREAST AND OVARIAN CANCER

Genetic susceptibility toward breast cancer has been primarily associated with changes in two genes called BRCA1 and BRCA2. In families with multiple cases of breast cancer, about half of the cancers can be linked to mutations of BRCA1, most of the rest to BRCA2, and some to a third gene called BRCA3 or to other presently undetermined alterations. Both BRCA1 and BRCA2 are quite long genes that appear to have roles in DNA damage-response pathways. BRCA1 mutations are highly prevalent in the Ashkenazi Jewish population. The presence of BRCA1 mutations has been linked to high mitotic activity, aggressive progression of disease, and a tendency toward negative hormone receptors.

Susceptibility to ovarian cancer may be increased as well. For individuals with these gene alterations, approaches to clinical management include use of magnetic resonance imaging (MRI), twice yearly breast screening, estrogen receptor modulators, and even prophylactic breast or ovary

36

removal. Germline mutations of other markers, such as p53, have also been associated with breast cancer development.

GENETIC COMPONENTS OF COLON CANCER

Dominant alleles have been identified for two types of colon cancer. Familial adenomatous polyposis (FAP) is relatively rare. Caused by an inherited mutation in the APC or adenomatous polyposis coli gene, it presents during childhood or young adulthood with copious (as many as 100) polyps in the colon. If these polyps are found by sigmoidoscopy, generally the colon is removed. However, drugs like sulindac have been used to arrest adenoma formation. Hereditary nonpolyposis colon cancer (HNPCC) is more common. HNPCC is actually a syndrome (known as Lynch syndrome) that causes a propensity toward the development of other cancers, such as endometrial and small intestinal cancer. Polyp development is minimal in these tumors, which are usually mucinous. The majority of mutations associated with HNPCC are on four genes called PMS2, MSH2, MLH1, and MSH6. Individuals under age 50 with colorectal cancer are usually checked for replication error repair (RER) mutations of MSH6. In HNPCC carriers, frequent screening colonoscopies beginning as early as age 20 are suggested. Women should also be examined for malignancies during pelvic exams or transvaginal ultrasounds.

GENETIC COMPONENTS OF PROSTATE CANCER

Development of prostate cancer is very prevalent in males as they age. Therefore, it has been difficult to identify possible genetic components of this disease. The BRCA1 and BRCA2 genes have been proven to enhance risk (moderately) for prostate cancer over the course of a lifetime. Other possible associations include mutations of another gene, HOXB13, various receptors, and more. A screening test for the presence of prostate specific antigen or PSA is more likely to be used to test for this disease, as PSA levels above 10 ng/mL have been correlated with the presence of prostate cancer. Caution in interpreting PSA levels is necessary, however, as infections, trauma, and other processes can produce transient PSA elevation. When PSA levels are persistently elevated, then the usual clinical course is transrectal ultrasound or digital rectal exam (DRE) coupled with needle biopsy.

GENETIC COMPONENTS OF MULTIPLE ENDOCRINE NEOPLASIAS

There are two types of multiple endocrine neoplasias, MEN1 and MEN2. Each type can present as several kinds of tumors originating from hormone-associated tissue types. Multiple endocrine neoplasia type 1 usually presents through parathyroid adenomas, possibly in conjunction with pancreatic islet cell tumors or other malignancies. Type 1 is linked to multiple mutations on the MEN1 gene. Screening includes checking hormone levels, proteins, pituitary size, and more. The most common types of tumors found in multiple endocrine neoplasia type 2 are medullary thyroid carcinoma and pheochromocytoma. A gene called RET appears to give rise to several classes of mutations associated with neoplasia type 2, including MEN2a (which includes the variant FMCT) and MEN2b. RET screening is the definitive diagnostic test. Prophylactic removal of the thyroid is recommended in these individuals.

GENETIC COMPONENTS OF MELANOMA SYNDROMES

Up to 15% of malignant melanoma moles appear to be associated with a familial syndrome. Many of these individuals present first with a highly pigmented raised or flat lesion called a dysplastic nevus. The syndrome has been associated with several inherited mutations, primarily in the CDKN2A gene and to a lesser extent in the CDK4 allele, as well as in a portion of chromosome 1p and the microphthalmia-associated transcription factor (MITF) gene. Not all linkages between melanoma syndromes and gene regions have been clearly identified. Therefore, genetic testing in this case has little prognostic value. Nevertheless, individuals with known CDKN2A mutations or a family history of melanoma should have whole-body skin inspections twice a year.

GENETIC COMPONENTS OF RETINOBLASTOMA

Retinoblastoma is the chief type of pediatric eye tumor. A portion of these tumors arising in the retina are hereditary in nature. Since retinoblastoma can develop at a very early age, knowledge of genetic predisposition and rapid diagnosis are both essential. Mutations in a gene called RBI appear to be associated with familial retinoblastoma. Even when these tumors are surgically removed as a child, an individual with a genetic component for retinoblastoma can develop a number of other types of tumors later in life, including sarcomas, brain cancer, and tumors of fatty tissues called lipomas.

GENETIC COMPONENTS OF NEUROFIBROMATOSIS

There are two types of inherited genetic mutations associated with neurofibromatosis, Neurofibromatosis type 1 (NF1) and type 2 (NF2). The first type, linked to mutations in the NF1 gene, is a disorder characterized by brown or café au lait skin spots and evidence of neural and connective tissue involvement, such as presence of neurofibromas and gliomas. NF1 carriers tend to develop other relatively obscure cancers as well. Management is difficult and swift detection and surgical interventions are the only effective options. There is another rarer type of neurofibromatosis associated with another gene called NF2. Tumors involving the nervous system including schwannomas, which affect myelin-secreting cells, may develop. They can be diagnosed during a physical examination when the malignancy pushes against the cranial nerve, causing hearing loss or a ringing in the ear. Surgery is the only effective management option, but mortality rates are high due to the nature of the malignancy.

GENETIC COMPONENTS OF VON-HIPPEL-LINDAU SYNDROME

Von-Hippel-Lindau (VHL) syndrome is the primary inherited type of adult renal cell carcinoma. It is very uncommon, but individuals with this syndrome tend to develop not only renal cell carcinoma but also other tumors, such as pancreatic cysts, retinal angiomas, pheochromocytomas, and hemangioblastomas of the cerebellum. The most common clinical features are impaired vision and frequent headaches, with typical onset during young adulthood. Inheritance has been linked to the VHL gene, and familial genetic testing is suggested for risk management. Frequent screening for evidence of the syndrome is also indicated, with regular eye exams, blood pressure monitoring, and ultrasound or CT scans of the abdomen or pelvis.

INHERITED VERSION OF BASAL CELL CARCINOMA

Basal cells are located in the lower layers of the epidermis of the skin. Malignant carcinomas derived from these cells are the most widespread type of skin malignancy. A subset of these carcinomas appears to have a genetic component, known as nevoid basal cell carcinoma syndrome (NBCCS). Individuals with this syndrome present with a variety of basal cell-derived carcinomas, especially on the skin and in the jaw area, and they are very vulnerable to ionizing radiation. These carcinomas often present at an early age, which indicates genetic testing. The genetic marker is the PTCH1 gene. The major management issues with NBCCS are either aesthetic or the possibility of malignant conversion. These types of tumors are not particularly life threatening and they do not cause premature death.

CARNEY COMPLEX

Carney complex is a condition characterized by the co-occurrence of many different malignancies. Abnormalities in skin pigmentation (including in the area of the vagina or penis) and benign connective tissue tumors of the heart, called myxomas, are usually observed initially. Since these myxomas obstruct blood flow, the possibility of death is a real issue. Primary pigmented nodular adrenocortical disease (PPNAD) and other endocrine tumors are often found in individuals with Carney complex as well. A little less than half of individuals with Carney complex appear to have an inherited component, identified as a mutation in the PRKAR1A gene. Babies with this gene should be tested by echocardiography to assess for myxomas. People with Carney complex should have annual ECGs and various types of diagnostic imaging tests to look for the possible neoplasms.

Cowden Syndrome

Cowden syndrome (CS) is a set of possibly malignant or benign tumors associated with the presence of two mutated alleles of the PTEN gene. The PTEN gene codes for tumor suppression via disruption of the cell cycle and/or apoptosis. Tumors of the endometrium, breast, and thyroid are the most common in CS. Genetic screening for the mutations is indicated. Clinical tests for the associated tumors should be initiated at much earlier ages than in the general population.

Birt-Hogg-Dube Syndrome and Rhabdoid Predisposition Syndromes

Birt-Hogg-Dube syndrome (BHD) is another autosomal dominant inherited syndrome encoded by the BHD gene. It is quite rare and presents with either light colored bumps in the facial or upper torso region, with air in the pleural cavity, or through the development of renal cancers. CT or ultrasound scans for renal tumors or lung cysts are indicated, as well as eye exams due to possible retinal involvement.

Rhabdoid predisposition syndrome is another inherited set of neoplasms linked to a gene called hSNF5/INI1. The syndrome is particularly associated with brain tumors in children.

Identification of Cancer Susceptibility Genes

Cancer susceptibility genes can be highly or weakly penetrant in terms of their ability to actually trigger disease. The first step in identification of cancer susceptibility genes is to map out the pedigree of families with familial aggregation or manifold cases of a particular type of cancer. In particular, families in which there are at least three first-degree relatives, three generations, or multiple siblings that have the same disease are usually selected. The utility of these pedigrees is greater when the cancer presents early in life and when the lineage of the cancer can be traced to one specific side of the family. Genetic analysis is then performed using genomic scans. This process is more fruitful when other known markers can be excluded or other cancer types are not superimposed. Sometimes segregation analysis is also done. In this approach, individuals with similar responses to a particular cancer are interviewed and included in the gene scanning.

Genetic Recombination and the Identification of Genetic Linkage

During the portion of cell division called meiosis, in which the nucleus divides and chromosomes are paired, **genetic recombination** or crossing over and reassortment can occur. Four chromosomal strands or chromatids are present; two strands make up one chromosome and two chromosomes are paired. The probability of genetic recombination is related to the distance between the genetic loci. Thus, if loci are on different chromosomes, there is virtually no probability of crossover. This results in a recombinant frequency of 0, and the areas are said to be unlinked. If, on the other hand, loci are close together on the same chromosome, crossover events or mutations can theoretically occur up to half the time with a frequency of 0.5 suggesting a specific linkage.

Genome-Wide Scans

Various types of genome-wide scans can be done to assess for genetic risk factors predisposing individuals to certain cancers. The basic purpose of each is to look for evidence of polymorphisms (different forms of various markers). Most of the laboratory tests that look for polymorphism

39

information content (PIC) use some form of gel-based separation technique. This is followed by a method of identifying or amplifying the separated markers and comparing them to commercially available markers run simultaneously. Southern blotting is a technique that uses enzymatic digestion of DNA coupled with gel separation, membrane transfer, and probing with radioactively labeled DNA probes to look for restriction fragment length polymorphisms (RFLPs). Polymerase chain reaction or PCR methods use amplification techniques. Recently, small repetitive nucleotide markers, called microsatellite-based markers, have been developed for use as probes with the different types of scans.

SCANNING FOR SINGLE NUCLEOTIDE CHANGES

Single nucleotide polymorphisms (SNPs) are changes that can be identified using specific techniques. Analyses of multiple SNPs can then be assembled to identify a haplotype or group of closely-spaced alleles on a single chromosome that tend to be inherited together. Large numbers of these SNPs have to be put together to produce a genetic map. The utility of using SNPs for mapping for cancer susceptibility genes is limited, however, because of the low incidence of these genes in the general population. Usually, better information can be gleaned by studying certain restricted populations with significant cancer propensities.

LOD SCORE

The LOD (logarithm of the odds) score is a measure of how likely two genes are to be inherited together based on their proximity to one another on a chromosome. The LOD score is a number derived from the calculated odds of two genes being linked. If the odds are found to be N to 1 in favor of linkage, the LOD is found by the equation $LOD = \log N$. To go in reserve and calculate the odds from the LOD, use the equation $N = 10^{LOD}$. For example, if the odds are found to be 10,000 to 1 in favor of linkage, the LOD score would be $\log 10,000 = 4$. Generally, a minimum LOD score of 3 (equivalent to odds of 1,000 to 1) is required in order to establish a link between two inherited genes.

NONPARAMETRIC ANALYSIS TO MEASURE GENETIC LINKAGE

Nonparametric analysis uses only affected individuals to look at genetic linkages. Usually, haplotypes are constructed using some sort of computer program. While these types of analyses are easier to carry out than LOD scoring, they are prone to certain errors. Other members of the family are generally not tested, and it can be difficult to correctly classify them in terms of specific diseases without individual diagnostic testing. Subject selection depends, to a certain extent, on current diagnostic testing regimens. Even so, these testing regimens tend to become better and more specific every year and thus can meaningfully influence the dynamics of the analysis.

USE OF TUMORS TO AID IN GENE LINKAGE STUDIES

Tumors can be used to **positionally clone suspected cancer susceptibility genes**. One way to narrow down the region of interest is to look for the loss of heterozygosity (LOH) by matching up restricted genomic areas from one person's normal cells and tumor cells. The portion where the heterozygous haplotype of the normal cells is lost in the tumor cells (leaving one haplotype) represents a potentially relevant site. Another technique is called comparative genome hybridization or CGH. Here DNA from the patient (subject DNA), normal tissue DNA (reference DNA), and blocking DNA (to suppress signals from repetitive sequences) are mixed together with tumor cells to measure the relative amount of hybridization between different sequences. CGH uses fluorescent markers to measure changes in intensity corresponding to the loss or gain of chromosomal sections in the tumors. There are reference tissue banks around the country that can supply specific tissues for comparison. Reference probes, such as sections of messenger RNA targeting DNA sequences, are also available.

40

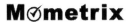

COHORT AND CASE-CONTROL STUDIES OF CANCER SUSCEPTIBILITY

There are two types of **clinical studies** used to look at the connection between candidate alleles for cancer susceptibility (or other associations) and the development of disease. The two, cohort and case-control studies, differ primarily in their method of subject selection:

- **Cohort studies** use the presence of a marker (or other exposure factors) to pick subjects, either prospectively (before cancer development) or retrospectively (after malignancies have been identified).
- **Case-control clinical studies** use smaller numbers of patients chosen on the basis of their disease status. Subjects are usually selected randomly from population sources, such as cancer registries. Alternatively, a portion of hospital patients with the disease and normal controls without the stated disease may be chosen. However, the latter process can tend to introduce bias into the study population.

Assessment and Diagnosis

BREAST CANCER PATIENTS
TYPES OF NON-INVASIVE BREAST CANCER

Noninvasive cancers are also called **in-situ cancers**. Within the breast, they are restricted to the ductal-lobular units and do not extend into the lymphatic or circulatory systems.

- **Ductal carcinoma** in situ is a stage 0 type of cancer. It is localized within the ductal-lobular units and does not extend into the bottom portion of the tissue. This type of cancer is considered preinvasive and women who develop this are more likely to develop invasive cancer in the future. This is usually detected through a mammogram and is not usually found on breast self-exam. It can be removed surgically.
- **Lobular carcinoma** in situ is usually not identified on mammogram or during breast self-exam. It is usually diagnosed as an accidental finding on biopsy of another lesion. The presence of lobular carcinoma in situ indicates an increased risk for invasive breast cancer in either breast in the future.

TYPES OF INVASIVE BREAST CANCER

Invasive breast cancer involves the breast tissue but also extends into adjacent tissues. This type of cancer has the ability to metastasize to distant parts of the body.

- **Invasive ductal carcinoma** makes up most of the cases of invasive breast cancer. It is located within the ducts but extends beyond the basement membrane to consume surrounding tissues. It may also travel through the blood or lymphatic systems.
- **Invasive lobular carcinoma** begins in the lobe tissue within the breast and invades surrounding tissue. Up to 10% of all invasive breast cancers arise in the lobe tissue.
- **Paget's disease** begins as a malignant lesion around the nipple and areola. The malignancy usually begins as a ductal carcinoma that spreads to include the external features of the breast. This form of cancer is usually very obvious to the patient because of the physical changes visible in the nipple and areola.

EARLY INVASIVE

The American Joint Committee on Cancer TNM Staging has recently developed a **complex staging classification for breast cancer**. In general, however, early invasive breast cancer would be Stage I or II (IIA or IIB). In these stages, there is either no lymph node involvement or only same-side axillary region lymph node involvement with no distant metastases. Nevertheless, diagnostic tests should include bilateral mammography (and possibly other imaging techniques), blood profiles, hepatic and renal function tests, serum alkaline phosphatase levels, and lymph node biopsy or mapping. Assays for prognostic factors like high levels of HER2 or hormone receptors may also be done. Management is surgery that either conserves the breast or a modified radical mastectomy in which the pectoral muscles are not removed. If there is nodal involvement or other factors exist (such as positive hormone receptors or large tumor size), adjuvant chemotherapy or endocrine treatment is added.

LOCALLY ADVANCED OR RECURRENT BREAST CANCER

Locally advanced stage III breast cancer is a comprehensive term for a highly heterogeneous grouping. All Stage III patients either have some sort of nodal involvement or their tumor has extended into the chest wall or skin. They do not have distant metastases. Once the disease has reached this stage, multiple treatment strategies are needed, including chemotherapy (and endocrine therapy in receptor-positive women), surgery, and radiation. Locally recurrent breast cancer, on the other hand, is generally due to insufficient removal of the primary lesion (such as with breast conservation surgery); it can often be managed with further surgery, although other modalities may be needed if there has been nodal or metastatic spread. Once there is metastatic involvement, therapies are merely palliative, and the prognosis is poor.

HISTORY AND PHYSICAL EXAM FINDINGS OF BREAST CANCER PATIENTS

Most patients with breast cancer do not have any symptoms. When taking a **history** from the patient with breast cancer, ask if they have felt a lump within the breast or axilla. If advanced, the patient may have noticed weight loss. Depending on the extent of involvement, there may be a noticeable change in breast shape. They may have noticed a discharge from the nipple when not lactating. If very advanced with metastasis, the patient may complain of back pain or other bone pain.

On **physical exam**, examine the breasts while the patient is sitting upright. They may appear grossly uneven or there may be dimpling of the skin present over the breast. With Paget's disease, the skin may have an orange peel appearance along with skin changes over the nipple and areola. A lump may or may not be palpable on exam. Clinical breast exam should include the axillae to check for any enlarged lymph nodes. The patient's weight should be assessed and compared with previous recordings, if available.

PROSTATE CANCER PATIENTS

HISTORY AND PHYSICAL EXAM FINDINGS OF PROSTATE CANCER PATIENTS

Patients may not have any complaints when they are diagnosed with prostate cancer. More often, they will complain of the same symptoms associated with BPH, or an enlarged prostate. There may be difficulty urinating because of the enlarging prostate applying pressure on the urethra. They may also complain of not being able to fully empty the bladder, frequent urination, or painful urination. If bony metastasis has occurred, the patient may have complaints of back or hip pain. At times, prostate cancer is not identified until a patient suffers a vertebral compression fracture, which is extremely painful and initiates imaging that identifies the metastases.

On **physical exam**, the patient may appear perfectly normal without any outward signs of the disease. A digital rectal exam (DRE) may reveal an enlarged or irregularly shaped prostate gland. If urinary retention has been a problem, the bladder may be palpable on abdominal exam. If advanced, the patient may have obvious weight loss or cachexia.

At present, about 16% of men will develop **prostate cancer** at some point, and approximately 20% of those will die of the disease. About 30% of men ages 30-40 have modest size prostate carcinomas. This percentage rises to about 65% for men ages 60-70. There are familial groupings of prostate cancer; for example, mutations in the RNASEL and MSR1 loci coding for host response to infection appear to predispose a man to prostate cancer. Diet affects susceptibility to prostate cancer as well; in particular, consumption of red meat cooked at high temperature to release aromatic compounds is highly correlated to the development of prostate cancer. Ethnicity may play a role, as African Americans in the US have an especially high rate of prostate cancer, but this may be due in part to diet.

DEVELOPMENT

Germline mutations in the RNASEL and MSR1 genes have been associated with an increased **risk of developing prostate cancer**. There is some evidence that inflammation and infection may play a role in the progression of the disease, and the development of lesions termed proliferate inflammatory atrophy (PIA) may predispose a man to later prostate intraepithelial neoplasia and prostate cancer. Molecular changes have also been closely associated with disease progression. These include somatic inactivation of the GSTP1 gene, which fosters susceptibility to oxidant and electron-accepting carcinogens, and depression of various functions caused by gene mutations, such as the PTEN tumor-suppressor gene, NKA3.1, and CDKN1B. As discussed previously, screening tests include serum prostate-specific antigen (PSA) levels and digital rectal examination. Diagnosis is generally confirmed by core needle biopsy.

LUNG CANCER PATIENTS

LUNG CANCER TYPES

There are three main types of lung cancer:

- **Non-small cell lung cancer** is further categorized as squamous carcinoma, adenocarcinoma, large cell, or spindle cell. The most common of these types is adenocarcinoma.
- **Small cell lung cancer** constitutes less than 20% of all incidence of lung cancer, but it is a more destructive type of cancer.
- **Mesothelioma** occurs due to asbestos exposure and is almost always fatal.

The presentation of lung cancer will vary depending on its location. A tumor located in the main airway, which is the most common, will cause wheezing and difficulty breathing. A tumor in the upper portions of the lungs can cause referred pain to the shoulder and down the arm. A tumor in the mid-lung may cause diminished breath sounds while a tumor in the lower lobe can cause a pleural effusion along with diminished breath sounds.

SMALL CELL LUNG CANCER

Small cell lung cancer (SCLC) is a rapidly-growing variant of lung cancer found in about 15% of new cases. Its origin is in the bronchi and this type of lung cancer occurs predominantly in smokers. At the time of diagnosis, the disease is usually symptomatic, and metastases have generally already occurred. There are 3 subtypes of SCLC: (1) oat cell or small-cell, (2) intermediate cell, and (3) small-cell combined with squamous cell carcinoma or adenocarcinoma. Differential diagnosis includes tests to distinguish it from slower-growing non-small cell lung cancer, lymphoma, sarcoidosis, metastases due to other primary tumors, or infectious processes. In addition to routine procedures like history, physical examination, and laboratory tests, SCLC is generally staged using imaging tests. In particular, a CT scan with contrast is done to assess the involvement in the lung

43

and other sites, and an MRI of the brain and/or a bone scan may also be done to look for metastases. A bone marrow biopsy may also be indicated.

NON-SMALL CELL LUNG CANCER

Non-small cell lung cancer (NSCLC) is a blanket term for several histological types of lung cancer not classified as SCLC. The major histological variants are adenocarcinoma, squamous cell carcinoma, and large cell. The large cell type is anaplastic, which means the cells are relatively undifferentiated. Diagnosis of NSCLCs includes exclusion of small cell lung carcinoma, metastatic lung lesions from other primary sources, sarcoidosis, and infections. The clinician generally stages the disease through use of history, physical examination, and laboratory tests. Imaging studies usually include not only CT scans but also positron emission tomography (PET), and, if metastases are suspected, a brain MRI and possibly a bone scan. Mediastinal node biopsies are generally performed if the PET scan indicates later stage disease; various types of incisions can be made, such as those into the sternum or mediastinum.

HISTORY AND PHYSICAL EXAM FINDINGS OF LUNG CANCER PATIENTS

When taking a **history** from the patient with lung cancer, ask about any smoking habits. This includes current or past tobacco use. Document tobacco use in pack years, which is the number of years smoked multiplied by the total packs of cigarettes smoked per day. A patient with at least a 20-pack year history is more likely to suffer complications from smoking. Also question the patient about exposure to any environmental hazards, such as asbestos, fiberglass, or coal. Obtain a thorough history about specific symptoms that are present and how long they have been present. Assess whether the patient has a history of other respiratory comorbidities such as COPD, asthma, or pulmonary fibrosis.

On **physical exam**, assess the patient's respiratory rate and pulse oximetry level. Auscultate the lungs and assess for any adventitious sounds or diminished breath sounds. Evaluate the patient for any sputum production with cough and assess its color and consistency. Examine the patient for any accessory muscle use with breathing and any signs of respiratory distress.

COLON AND RECTAL CANCER PATIENTS

Adenocarcinoma of the colon is usually slow to develop but can be more invasive than other forms of colorectal cancer. It is common to have metastasis to the lymph system with this type of cancer.

- If located in the **ascending colon**, the patient may experience a decrease in weight along with abdominal pain. When advanced, they may complain of diarrhea or constipation.
- When located in the **transverse or descending portion of the colon**, a bowel obstruction may occur. The patient may also experience a cramping pain.
- Cancers located in the **sigmoid colon** cause a narrowing of the diameter of the stool along with constipation.
- Cancers that form within the **rectum** usually cause bleeding and a feeling like the patient is not able to completely pass stool. They may also complain of rectal pain.
- Cancer in the **anus** can be adenocarcinoma, squamous cell, or basal cell. HIV patients may also develop Kaposi's sarcoma in this area. Anal cancers cause bleeding, pain, and the patient may notice a lump near the anus.

DEVELOPMENT

The factor most closely associated with development of colon cancer is age, with about 90% of cases identified after age 50. The vast majority of cases have not been correlated to any heritable gene mutation. However, there is a several-fold increase in risk of development of the disease when a close relative is affected, and there are several familial syndromes related to colon cancer (most notably familial adenomatous polyposis [FAP] and hereditary nonpolyposis colon cancer [HNPCC]). Risk of colon cancer has been associated with certain dietary practices, including high intake of low fiber and high fat foods. It has also been associated with environmental influences, such as exposure to tobacco. The disease often develops through mutations attributable to either chromosomal instability or to a lesser extent microsatellite (repetitive DNA sequence) instability. The genetic change most often found in patients with both precursor adenomatous polyps or actual colon cancer is a defective APC tumor suppressor locus.

HEAD AND NECK CANCER PATIENTS

Symptoms of head and neck cancer will vary depending on the location of the cancer.

- If originating in the **oral cavity**, the patient may notice redness or white patches along the gums, tongue, or oral mucosa. They may also complain of pain or bleeding in the gums, especially while eating or brushing the teeth.
- Cancers in the **nasal cavity** can result in upper jaw pain and headaches. The patient may also experience recurrent sinus infections or the feeling of always having sinus congestion.
- Cancer affecting the **salivary glands** can cause swelling along the jaw along with pain. The patient may also experience a numb sensation over the face or paralysis of the facial muscles.
- Cancers affecting the **oropharynx, nasopharynx, and larynx** can cause ear pain.
  - **Nasopharyngeal cancers** can also cause difficulty breathing and talking or headaches.
  - **Laryngeal cancers** can make swallowing difficult and painful.
  - **Neck cancer** will usually cause constant throat pain or hoarseness.

CERVICAL CANCER PATIENTS

When taking a **history** on the patient with cervical cancer, assess her family history for any relatives with cancer. Also ask about known infection with HPV or a history of abnormal Pap smears. Assess the patient's sexual history as well because HPV is transmissible from sexual partners. Any other cancer risk factors should be recorded, such as smoking.

On **physical exam**, the patient may not notice any symptoms until the disease has progressed. There may be a thin vaginal discharge present or some spotting after intercourse or between periods. They may also notice a change in their period with having it last longer and possibly have more discharge than normal.

Patients may have **complaints** of difficulty urinating or constipation when cervical cancer is advanced. This is due to the tumor tissue compressing the urethra or bowel. They may also complain of some rectal bleeding or visible blood in the urine.

OVARIAN CANCER PATIENTS

When taking a **history** from the patient with ovarian cancer, be sure to ask about any family history of ovarian cancer. There can also be an increased risk of ovarian cancer when a family member has a history of colon cancer because of similar tumor markers with CA-125. Ask about reproductive history including total number of pregnancies or any history of difficulty becoming pregnant. Question the patient about regular health screening habits, such as most recent Pap smear and mammogram and whether the results were normal.

On **physical exam**, the patient may or may not appear sick, depending on how advanced the disease has become. Early on, there may be some abdominal tenderness and vaginal bleeding

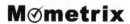

present. With advanced disease, a tumor may be palpable in the lower abdomen. The patient may have substantial weight loss, and the patient may develop constipation or an intestinal obstruction. Laboratory tests include a CA-125 which is a tumor marker for ovarian cancer.

TESTICULAR CANCER PATIENTS

Testicular cancer is more common in men younger than 35 years old. During the collection of **history**, questions should be asked to assess whether they perform regular testicular self-examinations. They need to find out if their testicles were delayed in descending as an infant or if they were present in the scrotum at birth. Another risk factor for the testicular cancer is the presence of supernumerary nipples.

On **physical exam**, a thorough genital exam will need to be performed. The size and density of the mass should be documented, as well as whether it can be moved or it is fixed to the surrounding tissue. Exam should include a rectal exam to assess for any changes in prostate size. Testicular cancer has an affinity for lung metastasis, so a respiratory exam should be performed to assess for any adventitious breath sounds. A chest x-ray should also be done to assess for any masses within the lungs.

BLADDER CANCER PATIENTS

BLADDER CANCER TYPES

The function of the bladder is to store urine before it passes through the urethra and out of the body. **Cancer tumors** form in the wall of the bladder and can cause bleeding because of cell damage. If large enough, a tumor can also cause a blockage in the urethra, which can affect voiding.

Most bladder cancers are described as **urothelial carcinomas** and usually appear in different locations within the bladder. These affect the epithelial lining of the bladder, and if metastasis is present, they can extend into the basement membrane of the bladder wall. Most of the urothelial tumors involve only the lining of the bladder wall and do not extend deeper into the tissue.

Papillary tumors are hereditary and specific chromosomal changes have been seen with this type of tumor. These involve the superficial lining of the bladder and the second layer of the bladder wall tissue.

HISTORY AND PHYSICAL EXAM FINDINGS OF BLADDER CANCER PATIENTS

Question the patient about the presence of any of the common risk factors for bladder cancer. Ask about previous employment and possibility of exposure to hazardous chemicals. Also evaluate the patient for any symptoms of dysuria, difficulty urinating, inability to urinate, or the presence of frank blood in the urine.

On **physical exam**, the patient may not show any outward signs of illness. If difficulty urinating has been a problem, an abdominal exam may reveal a palpable enlarged bladder due to retention. There may also be discomfort when examining the abdomen. The patient may also have an increase in rectal pain with firm abdominal palpation, if the tumor is compressing the rectum.

If the disease is advanced with metastasis, the patient may have visible weight loss or cachexia. Objective signs of pain may also be present with grimacing or guarding. Lymph nodes through the groin (inguinal) may also be palpable if enlarged.

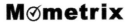

LEUKEMIA PATIENTS

CHILDHOOD LEUKEMIA

Leukemia is blood cancer in which white blood cells are overexpressed either in tissues or in blood circulation. The major mechanism appears to be acquisition of various genetic changes. Leukemias are classified according to the type of cell that is overexpressed and the acuteness of the disease. In children, leukemia usually presents as either acute lymphoblastic leukemia (ALL)—an acute increase in lymphoblasts, or acute myeloid leukemia (AML)—increased numbers of bone marrow-derived myeloblasts in the marrow or circulation. There are also a number of immunophenotypic subgroups of each based on antigen expression patterns. Leukemic children usually present with thrombocytopenia, anemia, neutropenia, and frequent infections and/or bone pain. ALL cells tend to infiltrate the liver, spleen, thymus, or lymph nodes. AML cells can accumulate in the skin, gums, and head and neck regions. Both types can invade the central nervous system. Exclusions in a differential diagnosis include idiopathic thrombocytopenic purpura, aplastic anemia, mononucleosis or other viral infections, rheumatoid arthritis, and small round cell tumors.

ACUTE LYMPHOCYTIC LEUKEMIA IN ADULTS

ALL comprises a smaller proportion of leukemia cases in adults than in children (20% vs 25%), and it has been shown to have some familial or inherited associations (such as a higher rate in twins or trisomy 21 of Down's syndrome). Two different viruses have been implicated in two variants of the disease—HTLV-1 for adult T-cell leukemia/lymphoma and Epstein-Barr virus in mature B-cell ALL. **Clinical findings** are usually vague symptoms associated with anemia, thrombocytopenia, neutropenia, and infection. On exam, enlarged lymph nodes and an enlarged spleen may be palpable. **Differential diagnosis** includes exclusion of other lymphoid conditions, infections like EBV or CMV, or metastases of other types of small cell tumors. Flow cytometry is usually employed to immunophenotype the cell lineage, because certain cytogenetic or molecular changes appear to be associated with a poor prognosis.

ACUTE MYELOID LEUKEMIA

Acute myeloid leukemia (AML) results from sequential genetic changes in hematopoietic progenitor cells or stem cells. These changes either inhibit differentiation or promote proliferation of the cells. Thus, exposure to known mutagens, such as ionizing radiation, benzene, or certain chemotherapeutic drugs can cause AML, and there are also rare inherited forms. There are four types of AML according to the World Health Organization, three of which incorporate specific sub-criteria, such as recurrent genetic abnormalities, multilineage dysplasia, or therapy-related myelodysplastic syndromes. The fourth category excludes these other categorizations. Cytogenetic subtyping is done because a poor prognosis or therapeutic potential can be related to the presence of certain markers. In particular, there is a subtype called acute promyelocytic leukemia requiring novel treatment with a regimen incorporating all-trans retinoic acid or ATRA. For all other types, patients are generally managed initially with anthracycline and cytarabine followed by further cytarabine or hematopoietic cell transplantation. The likelihood of complete remission diminishes with age. Acute myelogenous leukemia (AML) presents with generalized symptoms similar to the flu. Patients may complain of generalized achiness, fever, or fatigue. Symptoms may be more severe and include shortness of breath, weight loss, decreased appetite, vomiting, changes in visual acuity, and seizures.

CHRONIC MYELOID LEUKEMIA

Chronic myeloid leukemia (CML) generally affects older adults, with age at diagnosis usually over 60 years. Many patients either do not have symptoms or their symptoms are vague. Symptoms may include night sweats and low energy levels. The patient may also complain of left-sided abdominal pain or a feeling of fullness throughout the abdomen. On exam, the liver and spleen may feel enlarged. The patient may also have symptoms of a bleeding disorder due to decreased production of platelets. CML patients are often identified by an elevated white blood count (WBC) on routine testing. Blood counts and chemistries are essential in diagnosis, and other abnormalities of blood cells include basophilia, low numbers of blast cells, and often increased platelet counts. Splenomegaly is present in the majority of patients. CML is associated with the presence of the Philadelphia or Ph chromosome and a fusion gene called BCR-ABL, which produces a tyrosine kinase. These are tested for in suspected CML patients by either cytogenetic analysis or hybridization techniques, respectively. CML can be stable for a number of years but eventually becomes much more aggressive and deadly.

CHRONIC LYMPHOID LEUKEMIA

Chronic lymphoid leukemias are primarily B-cell lineage lymphoid disorders, with the most common of these leukemias being incurable chronic lymphocytic leukemia (CLL). CLL is diagnosed by the presence of more than 5000 mature-appearing lymphocytes per cubic mm of peripheral blood and a characteristic immunophenotyping profile showing expression of CD19, CD20, CDS, and CD23 antigens. Other leukemias and B-cell cancers must be excluded for diagnosis. Many patients are asymptomatic, or they may have lymphadenopathy or hepatosplenomegaly. Patients can be prone to infections due to hypogammaglobulinemia. Chronic lymphocytic leukemia (CLL) may present with the same generalized complaints as CML, but symptoms may be slower to appear. Once noticeable, the patient may have an enlarged liver and spleen on exam as well as enlarged lymph nodes. Symptoms of anemia and a bleeding disorder may also be present, necessitating a bone marrow aspirate or biopsy to evaluate treatment possibilities and a Coombs' test to look for autoimmunity. Cytogenetic analysis is useful but too expensive for routine use.

HISTORY AND PHYSICAL EXAM FINDINGS OF LEUKEMIA PATIENTS

When taking a **history** from the patient with leukemia, it is important to assess any past family history of cancer that may be present. Also question them about the risk of occupational exposure to radiation or chemicals, especially benzene. Patients with a positive history of HIV are at risk for developing lymphocytic leukemia that affects the T-cells. Also, patients with genetic diseases such as Down syndrome, Klinefelter's syndrome, and neurofibromatosis are at risk for developing leukemia.

On **physical exam**, the patient may have palpable or even visibly enlarged lymph nodes. If the platelet count is decreased, bleeding may be present at the mucous membranes, or bruising may be evident. The patient may also have frank blood present in the urine, or the patient may have dark, tarry stools because of occult blood. The patient may have an enlarged liver or spleen on abdominal exam. If the patient is anemic, they may be obviously pale, fatigued, or have an irregular heart rate.

LYMPHOMA PATIENTS
HODGKIN LYMPHOMA

Hodgkin lymphoma is a generally curable B-cell lineage disorder in which the malignant cell cannot produce antibodies, yet it does not die. The etiology of Hodgkin disease is unknown, but EBV virus appears to play some role. Distinctive Reed-Sternberg cells are found on biopsy. The immunophenotypic markers CD30 and CD15 are characteristic, but other antigen combinations are also present depending on whether the disease presents classically or in predominantly nodular form. The primary distinguishing clinical feature is lymphadenopathy in the supradiaphragmatic region. A modified Ann Arbor staging system is used based on radiograph, CT scan, and possibly bone marrow biopsy. Stage I indicates a single lymph node or extralymphatic site. Stage II means same side involvement but involving additional sites. Stage III designates malignancy on both sides

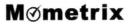

of the diaphragm. Stage IV is diffuse extralymphatic involvement. There may be no peripheral symptoms, but symptoms may include unexplained weight loss, night sweats and/or inexplicable fever bouts. Limited disease is treated with chemotherapy and involved field radiation. Advanced cases are managed with combination chemotherapy and multimodal therapies, including HSCT upon relapse.

NON-HODGKIN LYMPHOMA (NHL)

NHL is a blanket term for a variety of lymph node malignancies. Various leukemias or blood cancers could actually be considered lymphomas. Lymphomas can also present as solid tumors. The vast majority of lymphomas in the United States are of B-cell lineage, but about 10% are T-cell derived. Infectious agents, particularly viruses or retroviruses, have been linked to non-Hodgkin lymphoma. EBV virus has been associated with both Burkitt's lymphoma and large B-cell lymphoma. The presence of *Helicobacter pylori* has been linked to mucosa-associated lymphoid tissue or MALT. HTLV-1 has been found in adult T-cell lymphoma/leukemia. HIV patients may also have aggressive B-cell lymphomas. Pleural effusion lymphoma has been associated with HHV-8. Genetic abnormalities, altered immunologic states, and certain chemical exposures have been identified in particular types of lymphoma as well. Curability of lymphoma depends in large part on the etiology and site. For example, MALT is often cured through the use of antibiotics alone, whereas more intense therapies are needed for other lymphomas.

Screening and Diagnostic Techniques

FROZEN SECTIONS

Frozen sections are useful in the establishment and staging of a tumor when a decision as to the optimal type of surgical procedure is pending. They also provide information about the completeness of tumor removal post-surgically. They can elucidate the type of tissue involved so that it can be evaluated further, and they can aid in diagnosis through biopsy. However, the use of frozen sections is time-consuming and costly, so they should not be utilized when other options might be more complete or specific. Examination of the sections by a pathologist also has to be taken in context, because it is virtually impossible to examine every portion of the tissue. In addition, the use of freezing can damage tissue architecture and induce distortions.

IMMUNOHISTOCHEMISTRY

Immunohistochemistry (IHC) is a technique in which tissue antigens on frozen tissue sections are identified. The antigens are detected by the use of specific antibodies coupled to either fluorescent compounds or pigmented entities, allowing the pathologist to view these interactions on a fluoroscope or through a microscope. There are also various methods of amplifying the interactions, or enzymatically exposing masked antigens to aid in their visualization. IHC is used to distinguish between benign and malignant (antigen-positive) processes and to classify the type of tumor observed. It can also be a useful adjunct in determining the point of origin for the tumor and in identifying small areas that have metastasized. IHC can aid in the evaluation of the future aggressiveness of the tumor through the detection of characteristic nuclear antigens, and it can help predict therapeutic responses by identifying certain receptors, gene products, and proteins.

BIOPSY TECHNIQUES

Surgical interventions in cancer are based, in part, on information gleaned from biopsies, involving the removal of tissue for laboratory evaluation. At present, there are four ways that **biopsies** are obtained:

- **Needle aspiration**: The removal of tissue fragments through the use of a needle; this approach is usually highly specific and predictive if positive, but the sample size is typically too small to perform histological analysis.
- **Needle core biopsy**: Using a special needle to excise and retrieve a section of tissue large enough for histological analysis.
- **Incisional**: Surgical removal of only a small portion of the tumor; this approach provides more information but requires meticulous technique to avoid sampling mistakes and the induction of tumor spread.
- **Excisional**: Complete excision of a suspected tumor area; used for relatively small tumors or when other methods are inconclusive.

Most biopsies can be done with the patient receiving only local anesthesia, but general anesthesia may be required for excisional biopsies.

FINE NEEDLE ASPIRATION

In fine needle aspiration (FNA), a small gauge needle is used to extract cells from a tissue area that might be malignant, and then the cells are observed microscopically. The procedure is usually done before surgery and is attempted in conjunction with other tools, such as x-rays and laboratory evaluations. FNA is relatively non-invasive and inexpensive. The utility of fine needle aspiration is dependent on the nature of the mass because FNA can only broadly classify it and identify types of cells involved. Other issues, such as the architecture of the mass and its precise classification, are difficult to predict with FNA alone.

CYTOGENETIC ANALYSIS

COLLECTION OF SPECIMENS

Cytogenetic analysis combines the use of cultured tissues and various precise methodologies in the identification of chromosomal abnormalities. Tissue collection methods are designed to maximize the viability of the tumor cells ex vivo for analysis. Detailed patient information is sent to the laboratory along with the specimen, and the technician then chooses appropriate analysis techniques based upon this information. Usually a bone marrow aspirate (BMA) in sodium heparin is obtained for tumors of hematological origin; two to 3 milliliters of aspirate is generally sufficient. If it is impossible to obtain an adequate BMA (usually due to fibrotic tissue), peripheral blood samples or bone marrow biopsies may be taken instead. Other body fluids or tissues containing tumor cells may also be collected using sterile technique for cytogenetic analysis.

ANALYSES PERFORMED

Cytogenetic analysis is performed to look for chromosomal abnormalities during metaphase, the portion of mitosis where chromosomes align along an equatorial plane. Currently the following **types of analysis** are done:

- **Chromosome banding or karyotyping**: Uses techniques to visualize the bands between A-T and G-C pairs to search for abnormalities, such as translocations, deletions, and breakpoints.
- **Flow cytometry**: Looks for ploidy.
- **Fluorescence in situ hybridization (FISH)**: Uses fluorescently-labeled sequences of DNA to probe for complementary strands in the sample (a variant called multicolor or M-FISH uses several different labels).
- **Comparative genomic hybridization (CGH)**: Labeled tumor DNA is co-cultured with normal labeled reference DNA hybridized to standard metaphase chromosomes.

TYPES OF CHANGES IDENTIFIED

Cytogenetic analysis can distinguish whether chromosomal aberrations involve the following:

- No loss of genetic content but only relocations of DNA that give rise to different gene products
- Some deficit or gain relative to normal genetic material, such as deletions or duplications
- Amplification of genetic regions

Specific chromosomal abnormalities have been correlated with a variety of lymphoproliferative disorders and solid tumors. Any variation in the karyotype (i.e., the standard size, shape, and number of chromosomes) can also provide information about the prognosis for the patient by assessing whether the aberration is seen in a single clone of cells or in conjunction with other abnormalities in subclones.

FLOW CYTOMETRY

Flow cytometry is a method of analyzing populations of cells in suspension for various properties. The cells, such as tumor sample cells, are aspirated into the fluidic system of a machine called a flow cytometer. Here the cells are mixed with a fluid that places them in suspension, and a unidirectional or laminar flow is created. As each cell flows past a laser sensor, photons emitted are picked up and intensified by photomultiplier tubes. Data is electronically converted into either histograms or dot plots that compare characteristics of the cells in the population. In addition, fluorochromes are usually injected into the mixture in order to further highlight and identify the cell populations. A fluorochrome is a fluorescent dye, i.e., a substance that absorbs light at a particular wavelength but can emit it at more than one wavelength such as fluorescein isothiocyanate (FITC).

FLOW CYTOMETRY FOR ACUTE LEUKEMIA

Acute leukemia is one type of hematological neoplasia. Flow cytometry is used to establish the lineage or population from which the leukemia cells are derived, either myeloid or lymphoid. The most common approach is to isolate the blast cell population using a common leukocyte antigen called CD45 and then differentiate the cellular origin using other labeled antibodies. Flow cytometry can find and count blasts, identify the phenotypes of the leukemic cells, and pinpoint molecular or cytogenetic changes. It is also useful in the detection of minimal residual disease (MRD) in the bone marrow. MRD is identified in flow cytometry by utilization of a panel of antibodies that target antigenic markers that are expressed in different patterns in leukemic and normal cells.

FLOW CYTOMETRY FOR LYMPHOMA AND OTHER LYMPHOPROLIFERATIVE DISORDERS

There is no universal gating marker for B-cell malignancies such as lymphoma, so the initial step in flow cytometric analysis of lymphoma tissues is the segregation of the malignant cells using a general B-cell antibody like CD19 or CD20. The technique has limitations for lymphoma identification because these cells are difficult to bring into suspension, and fine-needle aspirates are often used. For lymphoma cases, tissue immunohistochemistry is often used in conjunction with cytometry.

On the other hand, chronic lymphoproliferative diseases are usually easily classified using flow cytometry. For example, B-lymphocytes found in the blood or bone marrow of individuals with chronic lymphocytic leukemia (CLL) express an antigen called CD38. CD38 levels are also prognostic for CLL outcome. Other B-cell disorders, such as hairy cell leukemia and T-cell disorders can also be characterized by flow cytometry, and MRD can also be pinpointed by the method.

FLOW CYTOMETRY FOR SOLID TUMOR ANALYSIS

At present, the use of flow cytometry in analysis of solid tumors is not standard practice in most institutions, though recent research has been directed towards expanding the possibilities of flow cytometry. If utilized, the technique is used to look for DNA content in one of two ways. DNA binds to a number of fluorescent dyes. The number of chromosome sets present, or the ploidy, can affect the peak distribution on cytometry. Another way flow cytometry is utilized is to determine the proportion of cells in the S phase where DNA is synthesized. Then that population can be examined. Even so, interpretation of cytometric data for solid tumors has not been as well defined as for the lymphoid malignancies.

MOLECULAR DIAGNOSTICS IN CANCER DIAGNOSIS

Various molecular diagnostic techniques are utilized to scrutinize the nucleic acid content or protein gene products in samples from cancer patients. Specific gene mutations have been associated with the presence of many cancers or their presumptive development. The initial step in all these techniques is extraction of nucleic acids by cell disruption. A fresh blood sample is preferable, especially if RNA or DNA content is to be assessed. This decreases the risk of DNA degradation. The anti-coagulants of choice are either ethylenediaminetetraacetic acid (EDTA) or citrate, since heparin can attach to nucleic acids. Some studies further suggest EDTA to be superior to citrate for plasma DNA testing. If fresh samples cannot be promptly analyzed, proper storage

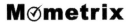

conditions are critical. Refrigeration for a few days is generally acceptable, and frozen, liquid nitrogen-stored, or paraffin-embedded older samples can sometimes be used.

MOLECULAR DIAGNOSTIC TECHNIQUES

The two most commonly used types of molecular diagnostic techniques are polymerase chain reaction (PCR) and Southern blotting:

- **PCR** amplifies the amount of DNA, which is usually then used in other methodologies, such as sequencing. An enzyme called reverse transcriptase is used to generate DNA copies called cDNA from an RNA template with short nucleotide chains or oligonucleotides as primers. The number of cDNA copies is then usually amplified through a process called nesting.
- **Southern blotting typically** uses enzymatic digestion of a patient sample, electrophoretic separation of the products, and then probing or blotting with suitable molecular probes. The latter methodology is labor intensive and slow.

There are also relatively new techniques using microarrays involving gene chips that arrange up to a million different cDNA or nucleotide probes in a pattern onto glass. Because this involves such a high number of probes, this technique allows for the quantification of certain DNA sequences within the entire sample.

ABERRATIONS IDENTIFIED FOR HEMATOLYMPHOID-DERIVED MALIGNANCIES

Molecular diagnostic techniques are sometimes employed as adjuncts to other tests for hematolymphoid-derived neoplasms. The typical gene rearrangements observed for B-cell or T-cell malignancies are in the IgH or TcR genes respectively. These rearrangements can be identified by Southern blotting or PCR. PCR is a particularly useful technique for pinpointing chromosomal translocations in tumor cells because of its sensitivity. Thus, PCR is often employed when looking for minimal residual disease. Molecular diagnostic methods are typically used before bone marrow transplantation, and utilize repetitive nucleotide sequences called simple tandem repeats or STRs to evaluate the likelihood of bone marrow transplantation success. The histocompatibility locus on chromosome 6 is targeted. In addition, any viral DNA which has been integrated into the nuclear material of malignant cells can also be detected by these methods.

DIAGNOSING SOLID TUMORS

A proportion of individuals with certain gene mutations are predisposed to hereditary cancer syndromes. Etiologically, only a few of these syndromes are localized in small genetic regions. Others are clearly more complex. Therefore, molecular diagnostic techniques are generally employed initially as screening assays for point mutations. PCR amplification is used in conjunction with either single-strand conformation polymorphism (SSCP) analysis or denaturing high-pressure liquid chromatography (DHPLC). PCR using larger probes, such as STRs, can be used to look for loss of heterozygosity (generally a deletion in the allele) in tumor cells relative to adjoining normal cells.

TECHNIQUES IN USE OR IN DEVELOPMENT

Many tumor-specific markers have been identified and more continue to be found. Knowledge of the presence of these markers in the blood or lymph can indicate metastases and aid in the determination of a patient's prognosis. Therefore, rapid PCR methods to detect these markers are in development.

Many other methods are currently available to identify proteins that are encoded by different genes and which may have cancer associations, including two-dimensional gels and laser techniques to excite the proteins. In the future, assays for methylation products of DNA and microarray assays identifying many of these expression products will become available.

TUMOR MARKER ASSAYS

Tumor marker assays quantify levels of certain molecules found in serum, other body fluids, cells, and tissues that have an association with the presence of malignancy. Most of the available assays are either radioimmunoassays (RIAs) or enzyme-linked immunosorbent assays (ELISAs), which respectively use radioisotopes or enzymes linked to various substances (often specific antibodies) as detection vehicles. The value of these immunoassays depends upon their specificity (i.e., their ability to accurately detect malignancy, versus normal tissue or benign growths) and sensitivity (the capacity for early detection during screening or preliminary diagnosis). The linearity of a test is important as well, as the concentration changes must be quantifiable and directly related to changes in tumor volume or response to treatment. At present, the measurement of cancer or tumor markers is generally more useful in the monitoring of disease, rather than in the initial diagnosis.

TUMOR MARKERS CURRENTLY USED

In order for a tumor marker to be a good candidate for a screening assay, it should be both organ and cancer specific. Some markers, such as carcinoembryonic antigen or CEA, are indicative of a malignant process, but they are not organ specific. In contrast, prostate specific antigen or total PSA is the ideal tumor marker for early detection or screening purposes because it is unique to the prostate. There is a range (4-10 ng/mL) where non-cancerous conditions, such as benign prostatic disease or BPH, can be picked up as well. When total PSA is combined with free PSA (which is lower in men with prostate cancer), the specificity of prostate cancer detection increases dramatically. Similarly, a carbohydrate marker called CA125 is a useful screening marker for ovarian cancer, if it is used in conjunction with other tests such as ultrasound. Thus, PSA and CA125 are valuable in screening settings, particularly if they show increases when measured sequentially. These screening assays are always serum or plasma-based.

DIAGNOSTIC AND PROGNOSTIC UTILITY OF ASSAYS FOR TUMOR MARKERS

Assays for tumor markers are generally more useful for disease diagnosis than screening, especially if they are used in conjunction with other types of tests, such as histology. Many of these markers are good adjuncts to tumor staging. Some of the more **useful markers** and their associated cancers follow:

- **CA125**: Useful for ovarian cancer diagnosis and monitoring in conjunction with other testing
- **Alpha-Fetoprotein or AFP**: Informative for distinguishing between various types of germ cell tumors, especially when used together with measurement of B-Human chorionic gonadotrophin (B-hCG)
- **Carcinoembryonic antigen (CEA)**: Can be elevated in colorectal, breast, and lung carcinomas; however, elevated levels are not tumor specific but can still be of prognostic or monitoring value
- **Tissue estrogen and progesterone receptors**: Have prognostic utility for the treatment of breast cancer, as test-positive individuals are responsive to antiestrogen therapies
- **Tissue HER-2/neu**: Useful in assessment of breast cancer patients for possible treatment with Herceptin

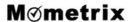

TUMOR MARKERS USEFUL FOR MONITORING SPECIFIC MALIGNANCIES

The following serum-based tumor marker assays are useful for monitoring the progression or remission of specific types of malignancies:

- **Prostate cancer**: PSA and prostate acid phosphatase
- **Breast cancer**: CA15-3, CA27.29, and for patients taking Herceptin, HER-2/neu
- **Ovarian cancer**: CA125
- **Pancreatic cancer**: CA19-9
- **Colorectal cancer**: CEA (also some limited utility for monitoring breast and lung cancers)
- **Nonseminomatous testicular cancer**: AFP
- **Thyroid cancer**: Thyroglobulin (contraindicated if the individual has autoantibodies)

Specific values are dependent on the immunoassay performed, so sequential values must be taken using the same test.

MONITORING DISEASE AND EFFECTIVENESS OF TREATMENT

The primary utility of most tumor marker assays is for the monitoring of disease progression and treatment effectiveness. After surgery, radiation, or other therapies, levels of certain markers should decrease within a few days if the treatment has significantly reduced the tumor burden. The lag time is dependent upon the half-life of the antigen in the serum and, sometimes, other factors such as renal clearance. If levels increase after treatment, then the therapy has not worked, and sequential measurements that are increasing indicate possible disease progression. International recommendations for monitoring intervals suggest samples be taken quarterly. If levels increase linearly, the time between samples should be lowered to every 2-4 weeks.

NONINVASIVE MEDICAL IMAGING TESTS

Any type of diagnostic or screening test is generally described in terms of its **sensitivity, specificity, and predictive value**. Sensitivity refers to the ability to detect small differences, and is defined as the percentage of positive test results in cases of true disease (when also accounting for false negatives). Specificity is the percentage of true negatives that are not picked up as false positives by the test. The positive predictive value is a measurement of the proportion of true disease positives that are detected by the test. In the case of **imaging techniques**, there are several ways of applying these concepts. Positive tests can be assessed on a per-patient basis in a population to evaluate the parameters of the test as a screening assay. The sensitivity, specificity, and predictive value can be evaluated within a single patient as well because they usually have multiple lesions or multiple areas with tumor cells. However, the predictive value of imaging tests is strongly biased by the size of the lesion (very small ones may not be identified) and the expertise of the radiologist or other specialist interpreting the image.

ADVANTAGES AND DISADVANTAGES OF USING IMAGING METHODS

There are advantages and disadvantages to the use of imaging methods for cancer detection. One advantage is that imaging methods are non-invasive. This can provide significant benefits in burdens, costs, and time. However, a key disadvantage is that tumor masses must be large enough for visualization by the imaging technique used. This is typically about 3-5 millimeters in diameter. Smaller lesions may well be missed. Other detection methods are theoretically much more sensitive. Cytology, for example, can detect a single cancerous cell. Realistically, however, laboratory methods usually only sample a small portion of the overall cancerous mass, whereas imaging techniques permit the technician to look at the entire tumor. Imaging techniques are also very useful in initial staging of the tumor and evaluation of changes after treatment.

IMAGING METHODS USED IN ONCOLOGY

The following types of imaging methods are currently used in oncology:

- **Traditional radiographs**: Uses x-rays and development on films (or digital methods); useful for detection of bone tumors and lung cancer.
- **Mammography**: As above, but with specialized machinery to detect breast cancer.
- **Computed tomography or CT scans**: Uses a rotating source of x-rays and image digitalization for greater clarity and multiple views.
- **Angiography**: Uses a vascular introduction of iodinated contrast media while taking serial images (generally digital); similar injections can be done with CT scans.
- **Ultrasound**: Utilizes high-frequency sound waves to produce an image; it is most effective in detecting malignancies in the neck and pelvic region or in the gallbladder and liver areas.
- **Magnetic resonance imaging (MRI)**: Uses an electromagnetic field, which excites atomic nuclei, to produce a digitalized image; used primarily for detection of tumors in the brain, spinal cord, and musculoskeletal tissues.
- **Single-photon-emission computed tomography (SPECT)**: Uses the injection of long half-life radioisotopes (primarily ^{99m}Tc) tracers to look at perfusion into bone or thyroid areas.
- **Positron-emission tomography (PET)**: Uses the injection of positron emitter tracers, usually coupled with agents involved with glycolytic metabolism.

DIFFERENCES BETWEEN IMAGING METHODS

Functional abilities can be picked up somewhat with modifications by use of ultrasound coupled with contrast media or MRI using spectroscopy at specific field strengths. A radiograph is the least sensitive modality in the group, and ultrasound and mammography are the least specific. Tomography techniques like SPECT and PET actually look at functional abilities rather than at anatomical features. They are very sensitive and relatively specific as well, especially PET scans. Recently, hybrid machines have been developed that can combine the functional capacities of SPECT or PET with regular computed tomography.

USING IMAGING BEYOND DETECTION AND MONITORING OF TUMORS

Information gleaned from imaging techniques can be used to design a therapeutic regimen. In particular, parts of the mass that contain biologically-active tumor cells can be targeted for introduction of radiation therapies. Different types of scans can be used as adjuncts during surgery to guide the surgeon. Modalities that are more functional in nature, like PET, have many potential applications, such as evaluation of the pharmacokinetics of therapeutic agents in the patient, tracking of stem cells, observation of the pathway that agents introduced follow, and the results of manipulation of these paths.

DIAGNOSTICS FOR SPECIFIC TYPES OF CANCER
DIAGNOSING BREAST CANCER

At present, about one in eight women is likely to develop breast cancer at some point. **Mammograms** or breast radiographs are recommended for all women starting at age 45 (American Cancer Society) to 50 (U.S. Preventative Services Task Force) every year or two. Starting at age 40, women should be given the option to get screened yearly, with a thorough explanation of the risks and benefits.

Mammography should be followed by **biopsy** if certain changes are observed. Areas of microcalcification or increases in soft tissue density on the mammogram indicate possible breast cancer. There are a number of other imaging techniques currently being evaluated as well, such as

MRI, PET, digitization of the mammographic image, and scanning with radionuclides. Clinical breast examinations can also distinguish breast cancer as firm, palpable masses that have irregular shapes. Breast biopsies are usually done by one of three methods:

- Fine needle aspiration followed by cytological studies
- Needle core biopsy along with either ultrasound or stereotactic direction
- Excision

For detection of primary breast cancer, mammography is the imaging method of choice. However, **other imaging methods** are sometimes used. For example, ultrasound is used to distinguish cystic from solid masses, and MRI with a contrast medium is used to determine the number of foci. Imaging can be particularly helpful in identifying which lymph nodes need to be removed if metastasis has occurred. For later stages, systemic metastatic involvement is usually evaluated with baseline bone scans and computed tomography of the abdominal and chest regions. PET scans might be used to look for metastases in soft tissues.

DIAGNOSING PROSTATE CANCER

It is recommended that men over the age of 50 undergo annual **prostate specific antigen (PSA) testing** along with a **digital rectal exam (DRE)**. Men with moderate to high risk of developing prostate cancer are recommended to get screened at ages 45 and 40, respectively. These two tests together can help with early detection of the disease. There is some controversy with this, however, because the entire prostate cannot be palpated through the rectal wall. Also, an elevated PSA does not always indicate the presence of prostate cancer. The test indicates that there is growth of the prostate gland, which can occur with benign prostatic hypertrophy (BPH) in the absence of cancer.

If DRE reveals a mass on the prostate gland, a transrectal ultrasound may be performed to differentiate between solid or cystic. A **biopsy** can be performed in conjunction with ultrasound to evaluate the tissue for the presence of cancer cells.

Once the presence of cancer is confirmed, **CT scans** and **MRI** will be performed to assess for any enlarged lymph nodes or metastatic spread to other organs. A **bone scan** will also be performed to check for bony metastasis.

DIAGNOSING LUNG CANCER

Lung cancer is usually discovered after a patient complains of a respiratory illness that lingers and a tumor is detected on chest x-ray.

- Routine **chest x-ray** may also reveal a malignancy that was previously not detected.
- Once a chest x-ray reveals a suspicious lesion, a **CT scan** is performed to further investigate the lesion and assess for any other lesions not seen on x-ray. Studies will also be performed on other organ systems to assess for metastasis.
- **PET scans** are performed to assist with staging the cancer.
- For definitive diagnosis and histological typing, **tissue sample** and **biopsy** will be performed. This can be accomplished with bronchoscopy, fine-needle aspiration of the lesion, or mediastinoscopy.
- Any lymph nodes that are suspicious will also be **biopsied** for the presence of cancer cells.
- If a pleural effusion is present, a **thoracentesis** will be performed to test for the presence of cancer cells.

DIAGNOSING COLORECTAL CANCER

Regular **screening** should be done to assess for the presence of colon cancer. This is accomplished through **digital rectal exams,** which allow the healthcare provider to assess for any masses within the rectum.

Sigmoidoscopy and **colonoscopy** can be performed regularly to assess for any masses or tissue changes that may be present. These studies are usually performed every 5 years, depending on the patient's history.

Biopsy of any suspicious lesions can be obtained during these studies.

Once a malignant lesion has been identified, the section of colon can be **resected** surgically. The patient may require a **colostomy** following surgery, which may be temporary or permanent depending on the extent of involvement within the colon or rectum. **Radiation therapy** can be done to shrink a tumor before surgical removal or can be done following surgery to ensure destruction of cancer cells. **Chemotherapy** can be given along with radiation treatments and is used when there is lymph node or metastatic involvement.

IMAGING METHODS FOR COLON CANCER DETECTION AND MONITORING

Imaging modalities are rarely used for the detection of colon cancer. Fiberoptic colonoscopy remains the method of choice, but virtual colonoscopies using **CT scanning** techniques are available. Non-invasive imaging techniques are often applied during colon cancer resections or for post-surgical monitoring. For staging purposes or monitoring, evaluation of metastatic involvement commonly includes CT scanning of the abdominal and pelvic region, the bowel, and the thorax (using contrast agents). **Chest radiographs** are sometimes substituted for thorax CT scans. Monitoring is usually done every 6-12 months, especially if CEA levels are increasing. In monitoring situations, **PET scans** are often the imaging modality of choice because of the increased sensitivity. Liver scans for metastases may also be performed using PET scans or possibly ultrasound.

DIAGNOSING CERVICAL CANCER

Pap smears alone are recommended by the ACOG for women ages 21-29 every three years as a screening tool for cervical cancer. Women ages 30-65 should have a pap smear and HPV test every 5 years. This test can also detect pre-cancerous cells so that early diagnosis and treatment can be accomplished.
- If a Pap smear shows abnormal cells, a **colposcopy** is performed. This involves applying acetic acid to the cervix and then performing an exam under magnification.
- If a colposcopy has abnormal results, a **biopsy** of the cervical tissue will be done. A cone biopsy is done if a larger section of tissue is necessary for biopsy.
- **HPV testing** can be done to test for a possible cause of abnormal cells on Pap smear. There is no treatment for HPV once it has been diagnosed; however, a vaccine is now available to reduce the risk of contracting the virus.
- If cervical cancer is diagnosed, a **CT scan** of the pelvis and abdomen will be performed to assess for free fluid in the abdomen as well as the presence of lymph nodes or other lesions.
- Other diagnostics may be performed to assess for metastasis.

DIAGNOSING OVARIAN CANCER

Unfortunately, ovarian cancer is often not detected until it has metastasized to other areas. In women who are not considered high risk, screening procedures are not performed. In women who are known to be high risk with a positive family history, **CA-125 blood testing** for tumor markers and transvaginal ultrasounds can be performed for screening. Ovarian cancer is usually diagnosed after a patient complains of secondary symptoms such as constipation or abdominal pain.

Laparoscopic surgery is performed to obtain tissue samples from the ovaries for definitive diagnosis. If there is free fluid present in the pelvic cavity, samples of this will also be obtained to assess for cancer cells. Once a diagnosis is established, testing is done on other body systems to assess for any metastasis of the disease. This will include **CT scans, chest x-ray, and bone scans**. If lesions are found on other organs, more tissue samples may be obtained to definitively diagnose the presence of metastasis.

DIAGNOSING TESTICULAR CANCER

Men starting as young as 15 years of age need to be taught to perform **testicular self-exams** monthly to evaluate for any abnormalities in shape of the testes or the presence of any lumps. A clinic exam should be performed on the genitals at least annually.

- When a lump is discovered, an **ultrasound** is done to determine whether the mass is cystic or solid. If solid, a biopsy of the tissue is done for definitive diagnosis.
- If positive for testicular cancer, an **orchiectomy** (removal of the testis) is performed. With the removal of only one testis, most men are able to go on and conceive children without difficulty.
- Studies will also be performed to assess for any metastasis of the disease. This will include **chest x-ray, CT scan of other organ systems, and bone scan.**
- **Renal studies** may also be done to assess for any kidney involvement.
- **Blood tests** to measure certain protein and hormone levels can also be performed. These may show some abnormalities with the presence of a testicular tumor.

DIAGNOSING BLADDER CANCER

Routine screening is not currently being performed for early diagnosis of bladder cancer. The disease is usually diagnosed after the patient complains of frank blood in the urine. Generally, the patient has no complaints of pain or other noticeable symptoms of malignancy.

- **Urinalysis** can detect the presence of blood. Specific studies can be done on the types of cells obtained through urinalysis.
- **Cystoscopy** can also be performed in which a thin catheter is inserted through the urethra into the bladder and a tiny camera is used to visualize the bladder wall. Tissue samples for biopsy can also be obtained through this test.
- An **IVP** (intravenous pyelogram) is used to assess whether the malignancy is located within the bladder or higher in the urinary system.
- **CT scan and MRI** can also be done to assess for the presence of tumors and to check for metastasis to surrounding organs.
- There is **tumor marker testing** available for patients who have a history of bladder tumors to assess for recurrence.

DIAGNOSING HODGKIN DISEASE, NON-HODGKIN LYMPHOMA, AND MULTIPLE MYELOMA

- Hodgkin disease is definitively diagnosed by performing a **biopsy** on the suspected lymph tissue. Cells are examined under the microscope for Reed-Sternberg cells.
- Non-Hodgkin lymphoma is also diagnosed through **lymph node biopsy**. Lymph nodes need to be examined microscopically to differentiate between characteristics of Hodgkin or non-Hodgkin disease.
- Multiple myeloma is diagnosed through testing that assesses the presence of **elevated levels of specific proteins** present with the disease. Electrophoresis is performed on both the blood and urine. With multiple myeloma, heavy-chain M proteins are elevated in the blood and light-chain M proteins are elevated in the urine. **Bone marrow biopsy** is also performed to assess for increased plasma cells.

With all three diseases, additional testing will be performed on other organ systems once diagnosis of the malignancy is confirmed. This includes **scans** of the abdomen, pelvis, thorax, and brain. **Bone scans** may also be performed, especially with multiple myeloma, to check for bone involvement.

IMAGING FOR LYMPHOMAS

Imaging plays an important role in the staging of **lymphomas**. Generally, computed tomography or PET scans of the pelvic and abdominal region are performed. After treatment, lymphomas often have lingering masses which may or may not contain tumor cells. Imaging techniques are valuable following lymphoma treatments because they can determine whether these residual bulks are actually viable. PET scans using ^{18}flurodeoxyglucose as a tracer will show increased uptake of the FDG if malignant cells remain. Depending on the treatment interval, this increased uptake indicates either a lack of response to therapy or a poor prognosis.

PRIMARY AND DISSEMINATED MELANOMA

Melanoma usually presents as a dark pigmented tumor visible on the surface of the skin, but it can also metastasize. Lymphoscintigraphy is used to identify lymphatic drainage routes that might provide a conduit for metastatic cells. If metastatic involvement is suspected, imaging techniques are used to locate the metastatic areas as resection of them may be possible. Typically, these tests might include CT scans (chest, abdominal, and pelvic regions), MRI imaging with and without contrast media, and positron emission tomography with the use of FDG as a tracer.

DIAGNOSING HEAD AND NECK CANCERS

Though there is no screening testing available, a thorough **oral exam** is recommended in patients who are at increased risk for developing head and neck cancers. This includes palpating the oral mucosa, including the area under the tongue, as well as assessing for any cervical and supraclavicular lymph node enlargement. If cancer is suspected, a mirror can be used to view the pharynx and larynx for the presence of any visible lesions. **Endoscopy** can also be performed to view the pharynx, larynx, and trachea.

CT scans are performed to assess for any tumors in the head or neck. This can also be useful in assessing for any lymph node disease or metastasis to other organ systems. If cancer is located in the nasal cavity or nasopharynx, **MRI studies** are preferred for more specific visualization of lesions.

Definitive diagnosis is accomplished through **biopsy** of the suspect tissue. This can be done by fine needle aspiration of cells or incisional biopsy of a tumor.

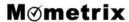

DIAGNOSING PANCREATIC, LIVER, AND OTHER TYPES OF CANCERS

The most common imaging algorithms for the remaining types of cancer are as follows:

- **Pancreatic carcinoma**: CT scanning with use of angiography
- **Liver cancer**: CT scans, CT angiography, MRI with the introduction of gadolinium; for primary hepatomas use PET with FDG for metastases from colon or other cancers
- **Endocrine cancers**: Depends on tumor site as follows:
    - Adrenal: CT using ^{123}I-meta-iodobenzyl guanidine
    - Thyroid: Radioiodine imaging (or PET with FDG if the tumor does not absorb radioiodine)
    - Neuroendocrine: CT with radio-tagged octreotide analogs
- **Esophageal and gastric cancers**: CT to stage, endoscopic ultrasound for invasiveness
- **Sarcomas** (soft tissue tumors): Usually MRI

Staging Guidelines

PROGNOSIS

Prognosis is defined as the likely course or outcome of a disease process. In cancer, there are many factors that can affect a patient's prognosis. **Type of cancer**, **location**, **stage**, and **grade** are all factors used in determining a patient's prognosis. The stage of cancer is directly related to a patient's prognosis. Often, medical staff use statistical data based on patients with a similar disease presentation to help determine a prognosis. Other factors such as the biological and genetic properties of the cancer cells may be used to determine prognosis. These "biomarkers" can be determined through laboratory and diagnostic testing. In addition, the age and overall general health of the patient are considered in determining prognosis. Patients with other comorbidities have the potential to have a poorer prognosis. How a patient responds to treatment is also a prognostic indicator.

TUMOR CLASSIFICATIONS

Tumor classifications include:

- **Carcinoma**: Cancer of epithelial tissue cells
- **Sarcoma**: A malignant tumor growing from mesodermal tissue
- **Lymphoma**: Cancer coming from the nodes or glands of the lymphatic system
- **Leukemia**: Cancer of the bone marrow stopping the marrow from producing normal blood cells
- **Myeloma**: Cancer in the plasma cells of the bone (Cancer in multiple bones is called multiple myeloma.)

ADDITIONAL DESCRIPTIVE TERMS FOR TUMORS

Additional terms used to describe the state of a tumor include the following:

- **Invasive**: The tumor can invade the tissues surrounding it by sending the cancerous cells of the tumor into the surrounding normal tissue
- **Metastatic**: Cancer cells from the tumor that have migrated to other tissues near or far from the original tumor
- **Primary tumor**: The original tumor
- **Secondary tumor**: Additional tumors that are composed of the identical tumor cells from the original tumor, that are transported to distant organs by cancer cells traveling through the circulatory system or through the lymphatic system

TUMOR GRADE AND CLASSIFICATION

Tumor grade is a description of how the tumor appears under microscopic examination. It is a determining factor in how likely the tumor is to grow and spread. Different grading systems exist for each type of cancer.

- **Well-differentiated** tumor cells appear the most like normal cells. These types of cancer cells tend to grow and spread more slowly. Well-differentiated cancer cells may also be referred to as **low-grade**.
- **Undifferentiated** cancer cells appear more abnormal and are associated with a poorer prognosis. Undifferentiated cancer cells may also be referred to as **high-grade**.

Based upon their microscopic appearance, pathologists can assign a numeric grade to the cancer cells. This information is then utilized by physicians to help determine the course of treatment and the patient's prognosis. Tumor grade is not considered the same as the stage of the cancer. Staging refers to the size and extent of the cancer and whether or not the cancer has spread to other areas of the body.

TUMOR STAGING VS. TUMOR GRADING

Tumor staging and grading are two types of tumor severity assessment. They are assigned by the surgical pathologist:

- **Tumor staging** is a measurement of the size or extent of spread of a tumor. It is based on three parameters, known collectively as TNM. There is also a distinction between **clinical staging** prior to treatment and **pathological staging** after surgical resection. On the other hand, tumor grading is a histopathologic evaluation of the extent of differentiation of the tumor.
- **Grading** assesses the difference between the tumor and the surrounding tissues. Grade 1 tumors do not differ much in appearance from normal tissue and are said to be well-differentiated. When the histopathological variation between normal and tumor tissues is large, graded as 3 or 4, the tumors are considered poorly differentiated (and more aggressive).

TMN CLASSIFICATION SYSTEM

The TMN classification system evaluates the stage of a tumor based on the size and extent of the **primary tumor (T)**, the involvement of **regional lymph nodes (N)**, and the presence or absence of distant **metastasis (M)**. If a system component cannot be measured, an X is placed after the letter, and a zero (0) is used for no evidence of that particular feature. The primary tumor, if it can be evaluated, is classified from T1 to T4 depending on its size or extent or Tis for carcinoma in situ. Regional lymph node involvement, if clearly present, is staged from N1 to N3 with increasing extent. Distant metastasis, if observed, is staged as M1 and the site is usually noted.

OTHER CLASSIFICATION SYSTEMS FOR TUMORS

Tumors are also classified in terms of their **histopathological grade (G)**, referring to the extent of cell differentiation in the tumor. If the histopathological grade is unclear, it is called GX. Otherwise, the grade is graded from G1 to G4 in decreasing order of differentiation. In other words, G1 tissues are well differentiated and G4 are markedly undifferentiated. There are other ways of describing the tumor. An **augmenting letter** is sometimes placed before the TMN stages for informational purposes (c for clinically increasing, p for pathologic, r for recurrence after period of no disease, or a indicating discovery on autopsy). The tumor can also be described by a staging grouping. The latter classification system has four stages: 0 for carcinoma in situ without other evidence of involvement, I for small primary tumor only, and stages IIA and IIB, which encompass a range of primary tumor and regional lymph node involvement without proof of metastatic spread.

PROSTATE CANCER

There are two staging systems that are commonly used for prostate cancer. The TNM system, which is adapted to many types of cancer, defines the primary tumor (T) when observable as T1 (identified only by histology or needle biopsy), T2 (limited to the prostate), T3 (reaches through the prostate capsule) or T4 (invasion of adjacent structures). The TMN system also expresses regional lymph node involvement from N1 to N3 and distant metastases as M1 if present. An X after the T, N, or M indicates inability to assess and a zero means no evidence of presence. The American Urological Association or AUA staging system classifies prostate cancer in four stages. These stages are fairly similar to the primary tumor staging of the TMN program. Basically, Stage A is disease that is not clinically observable. Stage B is a tumor confined within the prostate gland. Stage C involves malignancy that extends outside the prostate capsule but remains within the area. Stage D is malignancy with metastatic involvement. A Gleason score is a combined measurement of histological grading of the two most prevalent differentiation patterns; a lower score reflects a higher amount of differentiation and each component can be graded from 1 to 5.

BREAST CANCER

The most commonly used grading system in breast cancer is the **Nottingham grading system** (also called the Elston-Ellis modification of the Scarff-Bloom-Richardson grading system for breast cancer). This grading system evaluates the breast cancer cells on tubule formation, an evaluation of the size and shape of the nucleus of the tumor cells and the rate of cell mitosis. Each category gets assigned a score between 1 and 3, with 1 meaning that the cells most resemble that of a normal breast cell and 3 meaning that the cells are the most abnormal from that of a normal breast cell.

CERVICAL CANCER

Cervical cancer is screened for by pelvic examination, Pap smear, and possibly DNA testing for high-risk human papillomavirus variants. The malignancy is confirmed by cytology through either biopsy of gross lesions or colposcopy, and visual inspection of the cervix and vagina with a specialized instrument. These findings are confirmed by manual examination by the doctor and imaging studies. The disease is staged clinically by TMN-type criteria of the AJCC as well as the International Federation of Gynecology and Obstetrics (FIGO). Within the tumor size category T1 (or I by FIGO), which is basically cervical carcinoma confined to the uterus, there are subgroupings defined by degree of stromal invasion or size of visible lesion. Stage T2 (or II) is cervical carcinoma that extends beyond the uterus but not into either the pelvic wall or lower part of the vagina. Stage T3 (III) means that the pelvic wall or lower vagina has been invaded and/or kidney function is affected. T4 (IV) is further bladder, rectal, or extrapelvic involvement. Other distinctions like the N and M are standard.

UTERINE CANCER

The International Federation of Gynecology and Obstetrics (FIGO) stages endometrial uterine cancers either surgically or, if inoperable, clinically. FIGO surgical staging subdivides each stage from I to IV into various subgroups defined by increasing invasiveness. For example, stages IA G123, IB G123, and IC G123 describe tumor growth limited to the endometrium, tumor extension into less than half of the myometrium, or tumor extension into more than half of the myometrium, respectively. An earlier clinical staging format from I to IV addressed how far the malignancy extends. Surgery is done when possible and generally includes hysterectomy, removal of both fallopian tubes, lymph node sampling, and pelvic washings. Radiation of the pelvis and, if metastases are present, combination chemotherapy are also performed. Single modality radiation is reserved for patients with inoperable malignancies or symptomatic relief. Radiation therapy can be performed for tumors recurring after isolated surgical procedures. The prognosis is related to the stage of the presenting disease, its grade, and certain histological features like atypical hyperplasia. Major side effects of treatment are abnormal bladder and bowel function.

HEAD AND NECK CANCERS

Head and neck cancers are a diverse group of malignancies affecting the head and neck region. Head and neck squamous cell carcinomas (HNSCC) in the oral cavity, larynx or nasopharyngeal region represent the vast majority of these cancers. Some common presentations are hoarseness, difficulty or pain upon swallowing, or a referred earache. Lymphomas, sarcomas, and other solid tumors can also occur in this region. Head and neck cancers are typically staged by the traditional AJCC type of staging (TMN). A workup generally includes endoscopic assessment of the upper aerodigestive tract, regional imaging by computed tomography or MRI, a chest radiograph, and

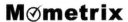

complete blood counts. Other imaging techniques, such as ultrasound or bone scans, are sometimes indicated as well.

CENTRAL NERVOUS SYSTEM TUMORS

About 85% of central nervous system tumors are intracranial in nature with the remainder arising in the spinal axis. Based on histologic features, the most common brain tumors in descending order are as follows: meningiomas affecting the meninges or membranes surrounding the brain (and spinal cord); glioblastomas arising from surrounding connective tissues; other astrocytomas, made up of star-shaped cells; neuromas, which grow from the nerve sheath; pituitary adenomas, from the pituitary gland at the brain base; and several other rarer types. Brain tumors comprise a small percentage of adult cancers but almost one-fourth of malignancies in children. The most prevalent brain tumors in children are generally treatable pilocytic astrocytomas and several types of embryonic tumors; medulloblastoma is an embryonic tumor occurring in the cerebellum. Advanced glioblastoma multiforme, which is a type of astrocytoma, occurs in about 4% of children with brain tumors and has an extremely low survival rate. Most brain tumors are located either supratentorially (overlying the tentorium cerebelli) or near the posterior fossa.

CARCINOMA OF THE PANCREAS

Most carcinomas of the pancreas are adenocarcinomas, and they are extremely lethal. Known risk factors include industrial chemical exposure, cigarette use, and chronic pancreatitis. Endocrine and cystic tumors each comprise another 5% of pancreatic cancers. If the tumor is situated at the head of the pancreas (true for the majority of cases), the patient usually presents with nebulous pain, jaundice, and weight loss. If it is located in the body or tail of the pancreas, then in addition to weight loss, the patient tends to experience either upper abdominal or back pain and may show signs of metastases. Staging of pancreatic cancer, which can usually be done using a laparoscope, uses typical TMN criteria with advanced T3 or T4 cancers extending beyond the pancreas. Triple phase helical CT scans are done, possibly in conjunction with other scanning modalities. Cholangiography (radiographic visualization of the bile ducts using contrast) is performed on jaundiced individuals.

COLORECTAL CANCERS

There are several classification systems for staging colorectal cancers. The most common scheme utilized is the Astler-Coller modified Dukes system. The emphasis of this classification scheme is the depth of tumor invasion into the colon wall. The modified Astler-Coller (MAC), the traditional Dukes, and the American Joint Committee on Cancer, or AJCC (based on TMN) classification schemes are interrelated. According to Astler-Coller, MAC A is comprised of lesions limited to the mucosa or sub mucosa; MAC B1 and B2 involve extension into or through the muscularis propria; MAC C1, 2, or 3 imply nodal involvement along with extension into or through the bowel wall; MAC D means evidence of distant metastases. These correspond roughly to Dukes' A, B, C, and D. The AJCC or TMN classification defines stages 0 (carcinoma in situ) through IV.

MELANOMAS

The severity of melanoma is primarily related to the thickness of the primary lesion and to the presence of histologic ulceration. The American Joint Commission on Cancer's Stage Grouping for melanoma reflects these parameters. The T or tumor size component for identifiable melanomas is up to 1.0 mm thick for T1, greater than 1.0 mm up to 2.0 mm for T2, greater than 2.0 mm up to 4.0 mm for T3, and greater than 4.0 mm thick for T4. Within each of these groups an *a* is added for no ulceration and a *b* is added to indicate ulceration. This is melanoma in situ. Regional lymph node involvement is described by an N followed by a 1, 2, or 3 (for 1, 2-3, or 4 or more involved lymph nodes) and an *a* or *b* to indicate either micro- or macrometastases. Distant metastases, if present, are classified as M1a, b, or c, depending on the site. As with other schemes, an x after the letter indicates inability to assess, and a zero means no evidence. Staging is from 0 (in situ) to stage IV (distant metastases). Stages I and II have no nodal or metastatic involvement, and stage III means regional lymph node presence. Within each stage I, II, and III there are various subgroups, and the presence of ulceration can put a thinner melanoma in the same stage with a thicker but non-ulcerated lesion.

HEMATOLOGIC MALIGNANCIES

The World Health Organization (WHO) initially separates or defines hematologic and lymphoid malignancies based on their cell lineage. For example, the basic lineage type could be histiocytic, myeloid, lymphoid, or dendritic. There are also subtypes within these lineages resulting in a total of 11 classifications. Each individual disease or syndrome within a classification is assigned an International Classification of Diseases (ICD) morphology code. Four of the groupings are **myeloid or stem cell conditions**:

- Chronic myeloproliferative diseases
- Myelodysplastic/myeloproliferative diseases
- Myelodysplastic syndromes
- Acute myeloid leukemias

Lymphoid lineage disorders are classified in the following manner:

- B-cell neoplasms
- T-cell and NK-cell neoplasms
- B-cell lymph proliferation of uncertain malignant potential
- T-cell lymph proliferation of uncertain malignant potential
- Hodgkin's lymphoma

The other categories are (1) histiocytic and dendritic-cell neoplasms and (2) mastocytosis, defined by increased numbers of inflammatory mast cells.

MULTIPLE MYELOMA

Multiple myeloma (MM) is a bone marrow disease characterized by the existence of single- or monoclonal proteins in the serum or urine, and amplified numbers of one type of plasma cell in the bone marrow, along with the formation of a myeloma or tumor composed of plasma cells and/or lytic bone injuries. **Multiple myeloma** is just one type of monoclonal gammopathy, or abnormal pattern of antibody production, comprising about 1% of cases; it must be differentially distinguished from other forms. Advanced MM patients tend to present with renal failure, advanced bone disease, high serum calcium levels, and abnormal cytogenetic patterns. There are a number of markers for poor prognosis, including elevated B_2-microglobulin, lactic dehydrogenase, C-reactive protein, and creatinine. There are three stages of MM with lower cell masses and urinary monoclonal protein and no lytic lesions in stage I, progressing to higher masses and protein and identifiable lesions in stage III.

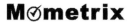

Cancer Survivorship

HEALTHCARE SYSTEM NAVIGATION

Patients with a cancer diagnosis must make many decisions about surgery, radiation, and/or chemotherapy, often with little assistance. Resources available to assist patients and families in **navigating the healthcare system** include:

- **Physicians**: The patient should go to the physician with a written list of questions about any issues of concern. Patients often become intimidated by physicians and forget to ask or are afraid to ask crucial questions.
- **Nurse navigators/Patient advocates**: Some nurses are specially trained to assist patients in understanding their options, making appointments, organizing lab and imaging reports, and finding resources.
- **National Cancer Institute**: The NCI provides extensive information about different types of cancer and current options for treatment.
- **Survivorship/Support groups**: These groups can provide emotional support and practical advice about dealing with cancer and the treatments required.
- **Community agencies/organizations**: Programs may be available to assist with meals, transportation, and lodging.
- **Internet resources**: Cancer.net provides much information about navigating cancer care for children and adults.

TRANSITIONING CANCER PATIENTS INTO SURVIVORSHIP PERSPECTIVE

Some of the most important aspects of helping a cancer patient into a **survivorship perspective** are educational. The patient may be provided with the following: documents explaining his or her present condition and prognosis; drug listings, including dosages and possible side effects; facts about the risk of secondary malignancies or other disease states; and detailed information about the appropriate healthcare professional to contact about various issues. The patient should be referred to support groups and to organizations focused on survivorship, and given publications related to cancer survival. A defined program that eventually weans the patient off dependence on the familiarity of office visits should be established. It is also beneficial to include rituals like a graduation after treatments are finished or an annually observed celebration of life.

SURVIVORS AND SECONDARY SURVIVORS

In the past, a survivor was the friend or family member who lost a loved one to cancer. They were the ones who cared for the patient and took care of them until the patient died and left them behind. Now, these caregivers and family members are called **secondary survivors**. The patient does not have to die from cancer for there to be secondary survivors.

The term **survivor** now refers to the cancer patient. The cancer patient is considered to be a survivor from the moment of diagnosis. Surviving cancer is now measured in the amount of time since the person has finished treatment or since they were diagnosed with cancer. Most healthcare workers refer to the survival of the patient in relation to 5 years. Often, prognosis of a disease is measured in the mortality rate from a certain type of cancer 5 years after diagnosis. A cancer survivor is considered a survivor their whole life, even if they have a recurrence.

STAGES OF SURVIVAL

The following are three different stages of survival and the nursing interventions that should be utilized with each:

1. The **acute stage** is the initial stage of the disease when a person is first diagnosed with cancer. Nursing interventions at this level are focused on education, which will continue throughout all stages. This includes education on the disease process, treatments available, and community resources available for support and further education, and the importance of compliance with the medical treatment plan.
2. The **extended stage** occurs after selected treatments are completed and includes the stage at which long-term therapy may occur. Nursing interventions at this stage are focused on continued compliance with any long-term therapy that will be started. This includes educating on the importance of continuing screening procedures to monitor for cancer recurrence.
3. The **permanent stage** is that stage in which a patient is considered to be cancer-free. This stage is reached when a patient is cancer-free for 5 years. Nursing interventions at this stage are once again focused on education, especially the importance of continued compliance with screening for cancer recurrence.

LONG-TERM PHYSICAL EFFECTS THAT IMPACT LIFE

There are multiple long-term **physical effects** that a cancer survivor may experience as a result of the cancer itself or its treatment:

- **Cardiac effects** such as heart failure, heart disease, and cardiomyopathy may occur, especially if a patient has received an anthracycline agent as part of their treatment.
- **Pulmonary toxicity** and inflammation of the lungs can occur as a result of chemotherapy (especially bleomycin), radiation treatment, or steroid use.
- **Endocrine problems** can occur after chemotherapy administration, hormone therapy, or surgery.
- Patients may have long-term effects on **fertility**.
- **Bone and joint pain** as well as **osteoporosis** can occur after administration of chemotherapy, hormone therapy, or radiation.
- **Nerve damage**, including peripheral neuropathy and hearing loss, can occur after chemotherapy.
- Surgery, radiation therapy, and chemotherapy can have long-term effects on **digestion and absorption of nutrients**.
- For patients who have had lymph nodes removed, **lymphedema** may occur, causing swelling and pain from the abnormal buildup of lymph fluid.
- Some cancer survivors may experience long-term **learning, memory, and attention difficulties** as well.

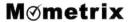

Employment Discrimination Laws

There are several laws that protect cancer survivors from **employment discrimination** related to their cancer:

- The **Americans with Disabilities Act (ADA)** and the **Federal Rehabilitation Act** are federal laws that prohibit employers from discriminating against their employees based on a disease or disability. The ADA prohibits discrimination based on genetic information related to a disease.
- In addition, the **Genetic Information Nondiscrimination Act (GINA)** also provides protection from discrimination of employees based on the results of a genetic test or a family history of a disease or illness. The GINA law covers the same employers that are covered under the ADA law (those with at least 15 employees).
- The **Family and Medical Leave Act** requires employers of at least 50 or more employees to provide up to 12 weeks of unpaid leave during any 12-month period to attend to their own serious health condition or that of an immediate family member.

Concerns Regarding Health Insurance

According to the Annual Report to the Nation on the Status of Cancer (1975-2012), 66% of people treated for cancer survive 5 years after diagnosis. Many cancer survivors experience financial hardship as a result of their treatment. Follow-up care for cancer survivors may include expensive testing and treatment to manage long-term side effects and potential disabilities. Some insurance plans will deny coverage for cancer-related illnesses if the condition is deemed "preexisting." Cancer survivors may have difficulty keeping and maintaining coverage. Resources such as prescription drug assistance programs may be of assistance for those who qualify.

- The **Patient Advocate Foundation** is a foundation that assists patients who have a chronic, life-threatening, or debilitating illness and may be experiencing difficulties with access to health care, job retention or discrimination, or a debt crisis related to their illness.
- **COBRA** is a federal law that gives an employee the right to choose to temporarily keep group health insurance benefits that would otherwise be lost due to a decrease in working hours, quitting a job, or loss of a job.

Financial Assistance Resources

Numerous local, state, and national organizations are available to provide cancer patients with financial assistance. Organizations include:

- **Patient Advocate Foundation**: Provides assistance for co-pays and transportation expenses for cancer patients and has aid programs specifically for those with metastatic breast cancer and multiple myeloma.
- **Partnership for Prescription Assistance**: Provides information about free or low-cost prescription drugs.
- **PAN Foundation**: Offers financial assistance to pay medical costs through 60 disease-specific programs.
- **Healthwell Foundation**: Provides financial assistance through the Emergency Cancer Relief Fund.
- **CancerCare**: Has a financial assistance program that assists with costs of transportation, home care, child care, and co-payments. Breast cancer patients can receive financial assistance for medications, lymphedema supplies, and durable medical supplies.
- **The Samfund:** Provides twice yearly grants to assist young (21-39) cancer patients with living expenses, tuition, education, medical bills, and various other health-related expenses.

69

SUPPORT SYSTEMS FOR CANCER PATIENTS AND FAMILIES

Patient and family support systems may vary widely and can include those that provide physical and emotional support:

- **Family members**: Family members (parents, spouse, siblings, children, grandparents) remain the primary support system for many patients and family, especially if they live nearby and can provide assistance although even distant communication can provide emotional support.
- **Friends**: Close friends may provide support in lieu of or in addition to family members and may, in some cases, be more aware of emotional needs because of longstanding close association.
- **Co-workers**: Co-workers may donate sick time, ease workload, and provide support in various manners.
- **Organizations**: Community organizations may help in provision of meals, transportation, visitors, and other types of support.
- **Religious/Spiritual organizations**: Some religious/spiritual organizations provide not only emotional support but also nursing care and financial assistance.
- **Online support groups/message boards**: Internet support systems, such as message boards for specific types of cancer, can provide emotional support as well as useful information on treatment and coping.
- **Support groups**: Local hospitals, senior centers, and organizations often provide a variety of support groups for both patients and family/caregivers, such as support groups for those with cancer.

TYPES OF CANCER SUPPORT GROUPS

Cancer support groups can take a number of forms. These may include the following:

- **Peer-to-peer groups**: These consist of individuals with similar cancer types and phase of cancer process.
- **Closed membership**: Structured groups meeting for a set period of time and restricted membership after initiation; the primary role is dissemination of information.
- **Open membership**: Meetings are unrestricted in terms of membership or time frame of attendance, there is flexibility about the issues addressed, and many include other family members as well as the cancer patient.
- **Background specific**: These groups are segregated by cultural or ethnic background or sexual preference.
- **Pediatric support groups**: Same age peer groups of children with cancer, their siblings, and parents are helpful but often not available.
- **Advocacy groups**: Factions focused on changing awareness, providing educational resources, and influencing political decisions and funding related to cancer.

Despite the improved quality of life shown to be associated with support group attendance, the majority of cancer patients do not attend any of these types of meetings.

SUPPORT PROGRAMS FOR SURVIVORS

There are many support programs specific to survivorship for people who have experienced cancer in their lives. **Cancer Hope Network** is a not-for-profit organization that provides confidential one-on-one support to cancer survivors at no cost. Cancer Hope Network utilizes volunteer staff that have also experienced cancer in their lifetime and matches those volunteers with clients who have had a similar cancer experience. In addition to the one-on-one support they provide, Cancer Hope

Network has a social network known as Hope Net that allows cancer survivors to create or join groups specific to their cancer experience.

The American Cancer Society and the George Washington University Cancer Institute collaborated to form the **National Cancer Survivorship Resource Center**. The program provides survivorship resources and tools to cancer survivors, caregivers, and health care providers.

SUPPORT PROGRAMS FOR FAMILY MEMBERS OF CANCER SURVIVORS

There are several foundations that offer support programs specifically for family members of cancer survivors. In addition, individual facilities in which the patient received cancer treatment may offer support groups or programs for family members:

- **The Angel Foundation** offers a variety of different camps, retreats, and support groups for family members of cancer survivors. They offer a free camp that is designed just for children who have a parent with cancer.
- **The Live Strong Foundation**, founded by cancer survivor Lance Armstrong, offers a multitude of services through its foundation for all cancer survivors, caregivers, family, and friends.
- The Live Strong Foundation has developed **Survivorship Centers** at leading medical institutions throughout the United States. These Survivorship Centers provide direct survivorship services as well as continue to advance in the field of cancer survivorship through research and the sharing of best practices.

COMMUNITY AND INTERNET RESOURCES AVAILABLE TO SUPPORT PATIENTS AND THEIR FAMILIES

Community and internet resources available to support patients and their families include:

- **American Cancer Society**: Provides support groups and assistance with non-medical expenses, such as durable medical equipment, transportation costs, and hair replacement wigs. The "Look Good, Feel Better" program provides assistance with techniques to minimize physical changes caused by treatment.
- **Group Loop**: Provides an online support group for teens living with cancer including discussion boards, personal blogs, and video journals.
- **National Children's Cancer Society** (NCCS): Provides financial assistance for non-medical expenses.
- **Ronald McDonald House**: Provides living accommodations for families, care mobiles, family rooms (in hospitals).
- **Sibshops**: The Sibling Support Project (amongst other organizations) provides workshops for siblings around the country.
- **Songs of Love Foundation**: Provides free personalized songs for children and teens with severe illness.
- **Starlight Foundation**: Provides personalized entertainment experiences for children with life-threatening illness.
- **13Thirty Cancer Connect**: Provides online support for teens and young adults.

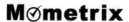

Cancer Recurrence and Secondary Malignancies

DEVELOPMENT OF SECONDARY MALIGNANT NEOPLASMS

ROLE OF GENETICS

A number of **genetic mutations** have been associated with the development of primary or secondary malignant neoplasms. The progression from primary tumor to a **secondary malignancy** after treatment is a complex process that is influenced by factors in the environment, lifestyle exposure to possible carcinogens, and various host factors, including genetic makeup, immune status, and hormonal contributions. Some cancer treatment regimens, when superimposed on these other factors, may induce the predisposition to development second malignant neoplasms.

ROLE OF CANCER TREATMENT

Surgery, radiation therapy, chemotherapy, and immunosuppression can all predispose patients to later development of **second malignancies**. Some of the more common possible second malignant neoplasms (SMNs) resulting from radiation therapy are thyroid carcinoma after neck irradiation, central nervous system malignancies like meningiomas or gliomas after cranial radiation, bone sarcomas in patients treated for retinoblastoma, and various carcinomas attendant to radiation therapy at a young age. Many classifications of chemotherapeutic agents have been correlated to an increased risk of SMNs, including alkylating agents, vinca alkaloids, epipodophyllotoxins, anthracyclines, topoisomerase II inhibitors and the steroid prednisone. The second malignancy is often a type of leukemia like AML, but there is some evidence that solid tumors may develop as well. There are also indications that the use of growth hormone in children may precipitate SMNs. Efforts to eradicate T cells in allogeneic bone marrow transplants have also been found to increase the risk of a B-cell disorder associated with Epstein Barr virus.

DEVELOPMENT AFTER RADIATION THERAPY

Radiation therapy has been found to contribute to the development of bone and soft-tissue sarcomas and a variety of soft tissue carcinomas. Data in many of the studies performed is hard to interpret because of other possible contributing factors. Some of the more interesting observations include an increased relative risk of developing breast cancer in the nonmalignant breast after radiation in younger patients (less than 45 years of age), an amplified chance of acute nonlymphoblastic leukemia after bone marrow irradiation, and high rates of second germ cell cancers in men receiving radiation therapy for testicular cancer.

DEVELOPMENT AFTER CHEMOTHERAPY

The majority of SMNs associated with chemotherapy for the primary tumor have been either acute myelogenous leukemia or non-Hodgkin's lymphoma. Many of the secondary AML cases occurred after alkylating agents were used to treat ovarian cancer, but other chemotherapeutic drugs have been implicated as well. There is some evidence of increased risk of the development of AML after chemotherapy for breast cancer as well. Studies have also shown increased development of later solid tumors in patients initially presenting with Hodgkin's disease who received chemotherapy, but otherwise solid tumors are rarely observed as SMNs.

ROLE OF SURGERY, IMMUNOSUPPRESSIVE AGENTS, AND HORMONES

The use of immunosuppressive agents or hormones to treat primary malignancies can precipitate second malignant neoplasms. Various studies have found an increased risk for the development of solid tumors, NHL, AML, MDS and skin cancer (especially squamous cell type) after the use of immunosuppressive drugs. Of the possible hormone therapies, estrogen has been most often associated with SMNs in both women and men. Radical mastectomies and lumpectomies have both been reported to contribute to the later development of angiosarcomas in the lymphatic system.

Tumors of epithelial origin have also been noted along the surgical stitching of ureterosigmoidostomies.

RECURRENCE RATES FOR COMMON CANCERS

Recurrence of primary cancer is a common fear for many cancer survivors. The chance of a cancer recurrence is dependent upon many factors, including the stage and grade of the cancer, the type of cancer, the treatment the patient received, and how long of a time period has passed since the treatment was completed:

- In **breast cancer patients**, the highest risk of recurrence is within the first 2 years following treatment. HER2 positive breast cancer is more likely to recur than HER2 negative breast cancer. Triple negative breast cancer is also more likely to recur in comparison with other breast cancers.
- **Colon cancer** is most likely to recur within 3 years of the initial treatment. The liver is the most common site for recurrence. The patient's age, preoperative CEA level, tumor location, size and cell differentiation, and the involvement of lymph nodes all play a large role in the likelihood of recurrence. The 5-year survival rate for stage 1 colon cancer is 74%, while the survival rate for stage IV colon cancer is only 6%.

Rehabilitation

REHABILITATION, ADAPTATION, AND REINTEGRATION

The aim of **rehabilitation** is the cure of the patient, or as near to that as possible, with the reinsertion of the patient back into his or her original environment with the same job, duties, and interpersonal relationships the patient had before the cancer diagnosis.

Adaptation of the patient is a consequence of treatment, with all limitations acknowledged and overcome to the fullest extent possible without compromising the patient's quality of life that was present before. The goal is to reenter life as before or as near to previous life as possible. There are many organizations that can give support and comfort, and ease the transition back into normal life.

Reintegration describes the process of assisting the patient to return to work through a program with their employers to understand each other's needs and how to work together to reach the goal of **re-employment**.

PHASES OF REHABILITATION

INITIAL PHASES

Rehabilitation is the systematic use of any measures that can restore physical functioning or address psychological or social problems in a patient. Typically, a cancer patient goes through several phases, the **first being the period when he or she is first diagnosed**. Here, the psychological shock of diagnosis is the primary target of any rehabilitation measures; for individuals with advanced disease, physical limitations may also need to be addressed. During the primary treatment phase, there are many sources of potential psychological or social problems. These range from toxic side effects from the therapy, such as hair loss and nausea, to anxieties related to treatment effectiveness and the inability to work or socialize as before.

PHASES AFTER COMPLETION OF TREATMENT

After treatments have ended, the patient transitions into a period where he or she recovers from the treatment side effects and returns to normal life activities and behavioral patterns. However, the patient is often still afraid of a recurrence. Later, the patient either moves toward long-term survivorship or recurrence and advanced metastatic disease. In either case, rehabilitative measures may be warranted. Long-term survivors can experience latent side effects, secondary malignancies, reproductive or sexual problems, and discrimination in the workplace. Individuals who relapse or develop metastases early on typically have new physical problems to treat, and they also have pressing psychosocial issues such as depression and dealing with probable death.

LONG-TERM FOLLOW-UP GUIDELINES FOR CANCER SURVIVORS

CHILDHOOD, ADOLESCENT, AND YOUNG ADULT CANCERS

The Children's Oncology Group (COG) has developed long-term follow-up guidelines for **survivors of childhood, adolescent, and young adult cancers**. The guidelines were developed with the objective of providing standardization and enhancement of follow-up care provided to survivors of pediatric cancers. The guidelines are evidence based and collectively compiled by a panel of experts with experience in pediatric cancers. The guidelines were most recently updated in 2018 and are available to health care providers who provide ongoing care to childhood cancer survivors. Each guideline is either based on the cancer itself or its treatment (e.g., surgery, chemotherapy, radiation). The therapeutic agent used as part of the cancer treatment is listed, along with the potential late effects the person may experience, risk factors, highest risk factors, the recommended periodic evaluation and health counseling, and further considerations.

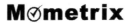

BREAST CANCER AND COLORECTAL CANCERS

The American Society of Clinical Oncology (ASCO) has developed guidelines for the long-term follow-up care of breast and colorectal cancer survivors. For breast cancer patients who have completed primary therapy with a curative intent, regular history and physical exams and mammography are recommended. During the first 3 years post treatment, it is recommended that physical exams be performed every 3-6 months. For years 4 and 5 post treatment, physical exams should be performed every 6-12 months and then completed annually (after year 5), post treatment. For patients that have had a breast-conserving surgery, a post treatment mammogram is recommended 1 year after the initial mammogram was completed and at least 6 months after the completion of radiation therapy.

For colorectal cancer survivors, ASCO guidelines state that a medical history and physical examination coupled with carcinoembryonic antigen (CEA) testing should be performed every 3-6 months for a period of 5 years. Computed tomography scanning of the abdomen and chest should be completed annually for the 3-year period after treatment. Surveillance colonoscopy is recommended 1 year after the initial surgery and then every 5 years after (depending on the clinical findings of the last colonoscopy performed).

POSSIBLE REHABILITATION ISSUES

PATIENTS TREATED FOR HEAD AND NECK CANCERS

In addition to the psychosocial problems possible in any patient with cancer, there are also site-specific issues for each type. Individuals with head and neck cancers who receive radiation therapy can develop dental problems such as tooth decay and osteoradionecrosis of the bone after treatment. Thus, they should see a dentist before surgery and be particularly attentive to oral hygiene afterwards. These patients generally require some type of supplemental feeding regimen as they may develop trouble swallowing. They often have post-treatment speech problems, as well, requiring consultation with a speech pathologist. In addition to speech therapy, some patients may also need some type of prosthetic sound generating device. Further, surgery may have severed the accessory nerve which innervates the trapezius muscle in the shoulder. If so, a physical therapist usually needs to work on restoration of the patient's range of motion. Lastly, cosmetic prosthetic devices must often be designed by maxillofacial prosthodontists for individuals with post-surgical facial deformations.

PATIENTS TREATED FOR BREAST CANCER

Regardless of the type of surgical procedure utilized, one of the most significant problems for breast cancer patients is post-treatment lymphedema, occurring as a result of axillary node dissection. If the edema or swelling is mild, it can be treated with measures such as salt restriction, diuretic use, elevation of the limb, and exercise. If it is more severe, compression sleeves or devices to normalize fluid levels are needed, and the patient is usually scanned for further malignant involvement. The patient may experience limited mobility and reduced strength in that arm. If a mastectomy was performed, the patient either needs a prosthetic breast or surgical reconstruction. Body image is a profound problem for many breast cancer patients, especially if the procedure was a radical mastectomy. They often develop psychosexual problems which may need to be addressed as well.

PATIENTS TREATED FOR PROSTATE CANCER

Men with prostate cancer tend to have many subsequent issues. Their cancer is usually diagnosed by routine PSA testing, which creates significant anxiety related to possible treatment scenarios. Further, any of the standard interventions can produce impotence, and pre-treatment sperm banking (if desired) should be offered to these men, as well as those undergoing treatment for other gonadal cancers. In addition, if the man has the carcinoma removed surgically, he can become

75

incontinent and possibly develop secondary rectal problems as well. If the treatment plan incorporates androgen withdrawal, he can lose his libido as well as body mass, predisposing him to osteoporosis.

AMPUTATIONS

Amputations related to cancer are most often performed in children and young adults, which mean that unique developmental, body image, and other psychosocial issues often need to be addressed. Relatively radical amputations may be necessary for patients with bone and certain soft tissue cancers. The physical therapist is important to these patients both before and after surgery. Before surgery, the patient is usually taught to walk on crutches, fitted for prosthesis, and anticipatorily prepared for the post-treatment plan. After surgery, the new limb can be attached when adequate healing has occurred, and at that point the physical therapist can begin teaching the patient to walk with it. There are also potential treatment plans that may save the limb, such as combination chemotherapy and radiation, especially for soft tissue cancers. Adequate information and counseling will be needed to aid patients in choosing between limb-conserving procedures versus the possibility of failing to fully eradicate the cancer.

End-of-Life Care

ANA CODE FOR END-OF-LIFE CARE

The ANA code for end-of-life care states that "the nurse provides service with respect for human dignity and the uniqueness of the client." It continues by asserting that "nurses individually and collectively have an obligation to provide comprehensive and compassionate end-of-life care which includes the promotion of comfort and the relief of pain, and at times, foregoing life sustaining treatments."

INTERDISCIPLINARY TEAM SUPPORT THROUGH END-OF-LIFE CARE

Members of the interdisciplinary team have vital roles in meeting the needs of the cancer patient during end-of-life care:

- **Pharmacists**: Provide guidance on medications, especially analgesia and antiemetics, including interactions and adverse effects, as well as dosage and equianalgesia.
- **Occupational therapists**: Can assist patients to compensate for physical weakness or deficits in order to allow them to remain independent in ADLs as long as possible.
- **Physical therapists**: Can help patients to maintain muscle strength and mobility and can recommend appropriate assistive devices.
- **Nutritionists**: Can provide nutritional guidance and assist patient and family in finding foods that the patient can tolerate and that do not exacerbate symptoms, such as nausea.
- **Spiritual advisor**: Can provide emotional support and help relieve anxiety as well as help the patient and family members communicate more effectively.
- **Psychologist**: Can provide the patients with tools to help to deal with anxiety, depression, and other responses to disease.

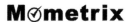

COMMON PHARMACOLOGIC INTERVENTIONS FOR END-OF-LIFE CARE

Common pharmacologic interventions for end-of-life care include the following:

- **Opioid analgesia**: Relieves pain and dyspnea
  - Risks: Excessive sedation, respiratory depression, constipation, confusion, myoclonus, itching
- **Antibiotics**: Reduce infection
  - Risks: Prolonged life and suffering, nausea, diarrhea, increased risk of *C. diff* infection
- **Oxygen**: Reduces dyspnea
  - Risks: Increases dryness of mucous membranes, interference with ability to communicate, depressed respiratory drive
- **Tube feedings/PEG tube**: Improve nutrition, hydration
  - Risks: Infection, local irritation, prolonged suffering, tube leakage, aspiration pneumonia, abdominal discomfort, gastric perforation
- **Mechanical ventilation**: Relieves dyspnea, prolongs life
  - Risks: Prolonged suffering, inability to communicate
- **Antimuscarinic agents** (glycopyrrolate, atropine): Reduces death rattle
  - Risks: Xerostomia, increased sedation, increased delirium
- **Glucocorticoids**: Reduces intracranial pressure, increases appetite, controls pain, reduces fatigue
  - Risks: Insomnia, GI upset, delirium, depression, increased risk of infection and hyperglycemia, Cushingoid syndrome, anxiety, increased risk of thromboembolism, myopathy, interference with other medications

NON-PHARMACOLOGIC COMFORT MEASURES FOR END-OF-LIFE CARE

Non-pharmacological comfort measures include:

- **Self-hypnosis**: Involves invoking an altered state of consciousness in anticipation of nausea and vomiting or pain episodes to decrease frequency, severity, amount, and duration of uncomfortable episodes.
- **Relaxation**: Progressive relaxation of muscle groups often involving imagery, which may be helpful to relieve chemotherapy-induced nausea and vomiting and pain.
- **Imagery**: Mentally removing the focus from unpleasant side effects and refocusing the mind on other images. It increases self-control while decreasing length and perceptions of nausea and vomiting episodes.
- **Distraction**: Diverting attention to other activities such as video games, puzzles, or humor.
- **Desensitization**: Involves relaxation and visualization to decrease perceptions of nausea and vomiting.
- **Acupressure**: A form of massage to increase energy flow and improve emotion.
- **Music therapy**: Often used with other therapies to influence physiological, psychological, and emotional states during and after nausea and vomiting episodes.
- **Positioning**: Allowing the patient to remain in positions of comfort, such as with head elevated, as much as possible. Turning and providing support to prevent skin ulcers.

ENVIRONMENT AND SPIRITUAL SUPPORT

Non-pharmacological comfort measures for end-of-life care also include **environmental considerations and spiritual support**:

- **Environmental considerations**: The environment should be maintained as quiet and peaceful as possible. Bright lights should be avoided. When possible, alarms on any equipment in the room should be silenced or turned to low volume. If a unit is noisy, closing the door and/or pulling bedside curtains may help to reduce noise and distractions. Chairs should be available at bedside for family members and visitors.
- **Spiritual support**: Kindness and compassion are essential elements of spiritual care. Patients' spiritual needs may vary, but all patients should be provided the opportunity to express their feelings and to have others listen, respond, and bear witness. The oncology certified nurse should help to arrange visits with priests, imams, rabbis, or other ministers according to patient's wishes and should facilitate spiritual procedures, such as healing ceremonies, blessings, and last rites.

HOSPICE

Hospice helps patients and families work through end-of-life issues while maintaining peace and serenity through the process. They provide medical care, self-care, supportive and emotional care, and bereavement counseling after a cancer patient dies.

Hospice services are available to those cancer patients who have a life expectancy of **6 months or less**. The hospice philosophy looks at death as another phase of life and a passage we all must go through. The goal is to make this journey as peaceful and comfortable as possible for both the cancer patient and the secondary survivors.

The hospice team includes a variety of healthcare providers from nursing assistants to doctors. Each person has a specific role to provide care for the patient and keep them as comfortable as possible. Many people are under the assumption that cancer treatments are not allowed when a patient is under hospice care. Chemotherapy or radiation may be continued as a form of palliative care to keep the patient more comfortable.

HOSPICE CARE NHO GUIDELINES

- The terminal prognosis of 6 months or less is determined by the attending physician.
- The patient and family or significant others are aware of the prognosis.
- Treatment is toward relief of symptoms not cure.
- The patient has had a progression of the disease.
- There have been multiple emergency visits or hospitalizations over the last six months.
- There has been a decline in the patient's functional status due to terminal illness.
- There are symptoms of impaired nutrition indicated by documented weight loss.
- The patient refuses further curative medical treatment.

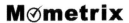

MEDICARE COVERAGE OF HOSPICE

Hospice is a healthcare program that provides support and comfort to patients and families dealing with the final stages of terminal illness. The goal is to provide care at home, although specialized hospice facilities exist in many locations. **Medicare** covers hospice care if all three of the following conditions are met:

- A physician certifies the patient is terminally ill with 6 months or less to live.
- The patient or family requests hospice assistance.
- The provider is Medicare-certified.

The physician's hospice referral can be made from either a home or hospital setting. To receive hospice care coverage, a patient must waive standard Medicare benefits for the illness/condition causing the hospice referral; however, care for other conditions unrelated to the hospice referral condition are covered by standard Medicare benefits. Medicare Part A pays for two 90-day and unlimited 60-day benefit periods, with recertification being subject to a doctor's (or nurse practitioner's) re-evaluation of the patient.

RESOURCES FOR LIVING EXPENSES, LODGING, AND TRAVEL

There are many agencies that provide resources for living expense, travel, and lodging for cancer patients.

- **Agencies** such as the Salvation Army, Catholic Social Services, The United Way, Jewish Social Services, and the National Association of Area Agencies on Aging have programs in place to help financially support cancer patients and their families.
- The **American Cancer Society** offers housing in **Hope Lodges** for patients undergoing treatment and their families. Hope Lodges are located throughout the United States.
- **Ronald McDonald houses** are also located throughout the United States and provide low cost or free housing to pediatric cancer patients and their families. Often, cancer treatment centers offer short-term housing options or discount programs for local hotels/motels.
- The **American Cancer Society** has a **road to recovery program** that assists patients with travel to their treatment center. Trained volunteers drive patients and families to and from treatment.

HOME CARE BENEFITS

Private insurance plans usually will cover some of the costs of home care on an acute basis; however, **long-term service benefits** may vary among different plans. They usually pay for skilled professional care services with the provision of cost sharing. Few private insurers may pay for personal care services. Most private insurers will pay for comprehensive hospice care. Some people have to buy Medigap coverage or purchase long-term care insurance to meet home care needs. Long-term care insurance originally protected individuals from huge costs that come with a prolonged nursing home stay. Currently, some long-term care insurers have increased coverage to include some in-home services.

KÜBLER-ROSS'S STAGES OF GRIEF

Grief is a normal response to the death or severe illness/abnormality of a patient. How a person deals with grief is very personal, and each will grieve differently. Elisabeth Kübler-Ross identified

79

five stages of grief in *On Death and Dying* (1969), which can apply to both patients and family members. A person may not go through each stage but usually goes through two of the five stages:

1. **Denial**: Patients and families may be resistant to information and unable to accept that a person is dying or impaired. They may act stunned, immobile, or detached and may be unable to respond appropriately or remember what's said, often repeatedly asking the same questions.
2. **Anger**: As reality becomes clear, patients and families may react with pronounced anger, directed inward or outward. Women especially may blame themselves and self-anger may lead to severe depression and guilt, assuming they are to blame because of some personal action. Outward anger, more common in men, may be expressed as overt hostility.
3. **Bargaining**: This involves if-then thinking, often directed at a higher power (e.g., "If I go to church every day, then God will heal me"). Patients may change doctors, trying to change the outcome.
4. **Depression**: As the patient and family begin to accept the loss, they may become depressed, feeling no one understands and overwhelmed with sadness. They may be tearful or crying and may withdraw or ask to be left alone.
5. **Acceptance**: This final stage represents a form of resolution and often occurs outside of the medical environment after months. Patients are able to accept death/dying/incapacity. Families are able to resume their normal activities and lose the constant preoccupation with their loved one. They are able to think of the person without severe pain.

SUPPORTING FAMILIES OF DYING PATIENTS

Families of dying patients often do not receive adequate support from nursing staff that feel unprepared for dealing with a families' grief and are unsure of how to provide comfort. Nonetheless, families may be in desperate need of this support from the nursing staff:

BEFORE DEATH

- Stay with the family and sit quietly, allowing them to talk, cry, or interact if they desire.
- Avoid platitudes (e.g., "His suffering will be over soon").
- Avoid judgmental reactions to what family members say or do and realize that anger, fear, guilt, and irrational behavior are normal responses to acute grief and stress.
- Show caring by touching the patient and encouraging the family to do the same (Note: touching hands, arms, or shoulders of family members can provide comfort, but follow cues from the family).
- Provide referrals to support groups if available.

TIME OF DEATH

- Reassure family that all measures have been taken to ensure the patient's comfort.
- Express personal feeling of loss (e.g., "She was such a sweet woman, and I'll miss her") and allow family to express feelings and memories.
- Provide information about what is happening during the dying process (e.g., explaining death rales and Cheyne-Stokes respirations).
- Alert family members to imminent death if they are not present.
- Assist the family in contacting clergy or spiritual advisors.
- Respect the feelings and needs of parents, siblings, and other family.

After Death

- Encourage family members to stay with the patient as long as they wish to say goodbye.
- Use the patient's name when talking to the family.
- Assist the family in making arrangements, such as contacting a funeral home.
- If an autopsy is required, discuss it with the family and explain when it will take place.
- If organ donation is to occur, assist the family with making arrangements.
- Encourage family members to grieve and express emotions.
- Send a card or condolence note.

Nurse's Role in the Final Hours of Life

The nurse and nursing assistant are an important member of the healthcare team throughout the process leading to death, and often develop significant bonds with the patient and family. Many patients and families prefer the presence of a nurse in the final hours of a patient's life, rather than a doctor, because of the close, consistent care-giving relationship. Some patients and families prefer to share those last moments privately. Accept whatever the patient and family choose. The presence of the nurse can be beneficial, as it provides the patient and family with immediate access to a member of the healthcare team who can answer questions regarding the actual process of death. The nurse ensures that everybody has a seat, points out where washroom, telephone, and cafeteria facilities are located, and offers to remain with the patient when family members need a break. If asked to be present, the nurse intervenes only as necessary, out of respect for the family's need for time with their loved one.

The interdisciplinary healthcare team prepares patients and their families for the **imminent death** of the patient. Nevertheless, the actual event is a time of great emotion. *If specific rituals cannot be conducted in a facility because they are against regulations, ensure that the family understands the limitations prior to the death.* Ensure that the patient and family are treated with dignity and respect prior to and after death occurs. Check the patient's vital signs. Record the time vital signs are absent in the patient's chart. If death occurred in a hospice, the nurse pronounces death. If death occurred at home, the CNA or nurse notifies the doctor, who comes to legally pronounce death and complete the death certificate. Do not begin post mortem care until after death is officially pronounced. Offer family caregivers the opportunity to assist in preparing the body if their cultural and religious traditions require participation in post mortem care. The body must be prepared before 2 hours elapse, when decomposition and rigor mortis start.

If it appears death will occur while the nurse is present, alert the family. Assist with contacting family members who are not present, and gathering those that are together. Be cognizant of visitors that are tiring the patient. Close the curtain around the patient for privacy. The patient is the top priority. Encourage family members to enter behind the curtain and speak to the patient singly or in pairs, if this is allowed under the family's customs and they wish to be present. Respect the family's specific religious or cultural observances surrounding the moment of death. If family members choose to remain outside the room, relay information to them as necessary.

Nearing Death Awareness

Nearing death awareness (**NDA**) is a common phenomenon among patients who are dying. When NDA occurs, the patient seems to be aware that death is imminent and may exhibit a sudden change in **mental status**, which may be dismissed as simple confusion. Patients may, for example, begin to talk about going on a journey or taking a trip. Others may say directly that they are going to die, or state a time, "I'm doing to die tomorrow." Many patients begin to talk about seeing or speaking to someone close to them who has died: "Mother is there waiting for me" or may report seeing "angels," "Jesus," "Buddha," or "heaven," depending on their religious beliefs. Some may report a bright light, report a feeling of peace, or report their mind is separate from their body. Others may stare into space and appear to be seeing or listening to something or someone although they can return to awareness if spoken to, so in this sense the experience is different from usual hallucinations. The **Greyson NDE scale** assesses this state with questions in 4 areas: cognitive, affective, paranormal, and transcendental.

ACTIVELY DYING

Active dying, or "imminent death", is defined by physical signs and symptoms that indicate likely demise within hours or days. Typically, the patient shows signs of profound weakness appear gaunt and pale, and the extremities are cool and mottled. He or she lacks interest in food or drink and has difficulty swallowing, which significantly decreases oral intake. Changes in breathing patterns are also common, including shallow respirations with decreased oxygen concentration, dyspnea, Cheyne-Stokes or other irregular patterns, and gurgling or gravely sounds in the back of the throat from excess secretions. There may be transient improvements in comfort, pain sensation and mental status, but the overall state is one of varying agitation, restlessness, delirium and confusion, increased pain, profound sleepiness, reduced awareness, difficulty concentrating and disorientation to time and place. A semi-comatose or fully comatose state may emerge.

The patient may also experience incontinence of both bowel and bladder. Third-spaced fluids may gradually be reabsorbed, decreasing the amount of swelling present. The pupils may become fixed and dilated.

FEEDING

A dying patient is not taking in **adequate nutrition**, so his or her metabolism changes and energy declines. When this happens, the patient will have less awake time, which can cause the family concern. Food is often associated with comfort. The family's inability to provide this comfort for their loved one can be a source of distress. The CNA or nurse can assist the family by educating them to the problems a patient may experience by consuming more than desired at this point. The dying patient's altered metabolism means his or her body is unable to handle nutrients in a normal way. Excess food and fluid will cause an increase in respiratory and gastric secretions that can result in dyspnea, abdominal distention, pain, and peripheral edema. All of these conditions put the patient at risk for infection, skin breakdown and pain.

PROVIDING FLUIDS

Most actively dying patients are **dehydrated** because they are no longer consuming adequate food and fluids, but there is little discomfort associated with this. Dehydration helps reduce nausea, vomiting, and edema for end-stage patients. The most common complaint is dry lips, nasal membranes, and mouth. Oral and nasal drying often results from increased mouth breathing, medication side effects (e.g., antihistamines), and supplementary oxygen delivered by mask or nasal cannula. The family may wish to provide the patient with fluids to drink as a way to relieve suffering and offer comfort. However, the result could be to increase the patient's distress by increasing respiratory and gastrointestinal secretions. Increased secretions lead to dyspnea, abdominal pain and distention, and peripheral edema. A bloated patient is at risk for skin breakdown, infection, and pain. Cleanse the patient's mouth and lips frequently with cool water or protective gel that help them retain moisture, to ease the discomfort without creating more problems.

EDUCATING THE FAMILY

It is often difficult for family members to cope with the physical changes associated with the dying patient. One of the most alarming is significant weight loss and muscle wasting, called **cachexia**. Food is associated with comfort and caring. When asking the family to withhold food, it can leave them feeling frustrated and unable to do anything to help. Reaching this point with the patient may force family members to accept that death is imminent. Educate the family about the physiological changes that take place in the dying patient to help them understand that the withholding of food is actually beneficial. The change in metabolism that results from decreased nutrition causes the body to produce and release endorphins, which are peptide hormones for natural pain control. Dehydration reduces the production and accumulation of secretions in the respiratory and gastrointestinal tract and reduces edema, and may decrease pain caused by the pressure tumors exert on surrounding tissues, all of which make the patient more comfortable.

CHANGES IN BOWEL HABITS

As patients approach death, it is almost universal that their intake of food and fluids decreases. Decreased input means **decreased output of urine and feces**. Monitor the intake and output of patients and be aware of the signs and symptoms of constipation and urinary retention. Constipation, abdominal distention, nausea, and vomiting can indicate bowel obstruction or volvulus (twisted intestine). Urinary retention can indicate kidney failure or a blockage from a stone or tumor. Diarrhea creates significant fluid loss and unbalances electrolytes; heart attack can result. Constipated patients are uncomfortable and more difficult to manage. Follow instructions in the care plan for the treatment of constipation.

CONGESTION

Patients experience **increased respiratory secretions** as they approach death, and are unable to clear them independently. Many experience a drowning sensation. Frequent episodes of coughing leave patients fatigued. Assist the patient with dyspnea to clear the airway by repositioning, and encourage deep breathing and coughing exercises. Use caution, because patients with osteoporosis may fracture ribs if they cough hard. Note the quality of the patient's cough – dry and non-productive, or wet and productive. The RN may suction the airway, and ask the doctor to prescribe antihistamines and decongestants. If the patient has a productive cough, the doctor may order the nurse or CNA to assist the patient to collect a sputum sample. The best time of collection is when the patient awakes in the morning, because fluid collects overnight. Wear gloves. Label the jar in ink. Open the sterile jar and ask the patient to expel lung fluid into it, *not saliva*. Cap the jar, place it in a biohazard bag, and refrigerate until pick-up by the lab.

INCREASED SLEEPINESS

During the last four weeks of life, end-stage patients experience a marked increase in **sleepiness** due to decreased intake of calories, dehydration, hypoxia, psychological withdrawal, organ failure, and vital exhaustion. As caloric intake decreases, the body conserves energy and shunts blood flow from the periphery to the core to preserve the vital organs (brain, heart, lungs, and kidneys). Rerouting the blood supply triggers the brain to decrease the amount of time a patient is awake. Depending on the underlying disease process, the amount of awake time a patient experiences may be related to a significant decrease in oxygen availability. A low blood oxygen level (hypoxia) will result in sleepiness. For those patients receiving opiates, an increase in sleepiness occurs as a side effect of the medication. Azotemia (also called uremia) causes sleepiness as the kidneys fail. Azotemia causes death 8—12 days after a patient decides to stop dialysis. Report increased sleepiness and changes in sleep patterns to the Registered Nurse.

AGITATION OR RESTLESSNESS

Patients experience **acute agitation** from urinary retention, constipation, dyspnea, medication side effects, and pain over the course of their diseases. When death is imminent in one or two days, many patients experience another final flare of agitation, which is difficult for families and caregivers to watch. It is the responsibility of the hospice team to monitor the patient for signs of agitation and be prepared with appropriate interventions. The most common cause of agitation in the dying patient is pain. If the patient is nonverbal, rely on physical symptoms to determine when the patient is experiencing pain. Reposition the patient. Monitor for signs that the patient needs pain medication. Divert the patient's attention through music or reading. If the patient approaches death with fear or spiritual unrest, it may express itself as agitation. Ask if he or she wants to speak to a chaplain. Chaplains have contacts among many religions, and can arrange visits from the appropriate spiritual leader.

WHEN DEATH IS IMMINENT

It is important that the nurse and nursing assistant to understand the cultural and religious beliefs of the patient and his or her family, because these two aspects are highlighted when death is approaching. It is the responsibility of the hospice/palliative care team to support the patient and family and to respect the wishes of the patient. The patient must be monitored for physiological signs that indicate death is imminent, even if the patient does not complain of symptoms. Most patients, within the last four weeks of life, will experience significant fatigue and weakness and require additional assistance. Pain may increase in the dying patient, or the patient's requirement for pain control medication may decrease as the body releases endorphins. Endorphins are polypeptide hormones produced by the pituitary gland and hypothalamus in the brain that act as natural pain suppressants. Most patients experience difficulty breathing (dyspnea) and this is most distressing for families. Careful positioning of the patient and improving air circulation facilitates breathing.

USE OF AIR CIRCULATION

One of the most common symptoms at the end of life is difficulty breathing (dyspnea). While this can be related to the underlying disease process, most patients near death experience dyspnea as a result of:

- Increased respiratory secretions.
- Increased breathing muscle weakness.
- Decreased ability to clear respiratory secretions.
- Metabolic changes that alter the effectiveness of gas exchange in the lungs.

Dyspnea is often the most distressing of symptoms, as the patient fears the sensation of suffocating, and the family is concerned because they are unable to provide relief and comfort to their loved one. The easiest and least invasive way for the nurse and nursing assistant to relieve dyspnea is to use fans to increase the **circulation of air** in the patient's room. Many patients report a decrease in dyspnea when they feel air moving across their faces. If fans are ineffective, inform the respiratory therapist or doctor that supplemental oxygen seems indicated.

PATIENTS' BELIEF SYSTEM

Often, patients approaching death feel they have lost control of their lives, which can be as distressing as their physical symptoms. The hospice/palliative care team must understand the cultural, gender and religious beliefs of patients and their families. **Belief systems** play a vital role in the expectations of the patient and family members. It is also important that the nurse/nursing assistant recognizes his or her own personal beliefs surrounding death, and does not impose his or her own belief system on the patient and family. Most patients find familiar family and/or religious objects comforting. Treat religious and family artifacts with the utmost respect. Regardless of where the patient is receiving hospice care, he or she deserves to spend time in an environment tailored to his or her preferences. A home-like environment provides comfort and security. Allow the patient to reach the end of life in peace, even if those his or her choices are not shared.

The nurse and nursing assistant must accept how **cultural and religious beliefs** of the patient and family require environmental changes as death nears. They may be required to place particular objects of sentimental value or religious significance around the sick room. The schedule may change to allow for religious rites. They may be asked to assist with ritual washing and dressing. Some patients prefer quiet and few visitors. If the patient prefers to be surrounded by family and friends, the nurse must rearrange the sick room to ensure the patient's privacy when performing personal care. Support the patient's choice of environment, whether hospice and palliative care is being given in a facility or the patient's home. Develop strategies so that the patient's choices do not interfere with those of other dying patients, such as encouraging the use of headphones. Examine one's own belief systems surrounding death and do not impose personal beliefs or preferences on the patient's environment. Respect the wishes of the patient and attempt to provide the environment the patient desires.

CULTURAL INFLUENCES ON NUTRITION AND HYDRATION AT END OF LIFE

Most cultures attach significant importance to the **role of consuming meals together**. As patients experience the progression of disease and approach death, the goals of nutrition and hydration change. Changing feeding routines often proves distressing for patients and their families. It is the responsibility of the nurse/nursing assistant to understand the changes and help support the patient and their family as the need for food decreases. As death approaches, the goal of eating and drinking is no longer to meet the nutritional needs of the patient. In fact, introducing food and/or fluids as the patient's organs shut down can cause or increase discomfort for the patient. End-stage patients produce increased mucous in the respiratory tract, which leads to dyspnea and the death rattle. If fluids are introduced, the body uses it to increase secretions, which causes increased respiratory difficulty. A more appropriate use of fluid is to moisten the patient's mouth for speaking.

Most cultures attach significant social importance to eating meals together and the hospice/palliative care team must understand the cultural background and the significance of sharing meals in that culture. As a patient approaches death, the goal of eating and drinking becomes social, rather than meeting the diminished nutritional needs of the patient. Anorexia in the patient signals that the dying process has begun. Families often exhibit distress because they perceive that the patient is starving. It is important that the nurse/nursing assistant understands the metabolic changes occurring in the patient's body, and educates and supports the patient and family. Patients who continue to consume food after metabolic changes have started organ shutdown will experience increased edema and discomfort. End-stage patients are unable to process food comfortably, as the intestinal tract slows significantly or stops functioning altogether.

PROVIDING COMFORT MEASURES AND DIGNITY AT TIME OF DEATH

The nurse should prepare family and friends for the changes they will see as the patient nears death and provide guidance in **comfort measures** for the dying patient:

- Ensuring pain is managed adequately, including medications, such as analgesics and muscle relaxants (if the patient is having muscle spasms), and complementary therapies, such as massage, Reiki, and music therapy.
- Providing mouth care with premoistened swabs.
- Gently washing and moisturizing the patient's skin with a warm cloth if the patient is cold and cool cloth if feverish.
- Talking softly to the patient even if the patient appears to be in a coma and non-responsive.
- Accepting and not challenging if the patient appears to be seeing or communicating with deceased loved-ones.
- Using FaceTime or Skype to allow family/friends who are not present to participate.

After the patient has died, some people will want to spend time sitting with the body and may want to participate in washing and dressing the body, and the nurse should respect their wishes.

POSTMORTEM CARE AND SERVICES

POSTMORTEM DECOMPOSITION

The process of postmortem decomposition begins almost immediately after death. **Liver mortis** occurs as the blood vessels become more permeable and red blood cells begin to break down, resulting in the pooling of blood and staining of tissue that occurs in dependent parts of the body (**lividity**). The skin may appear splotchy within 4 to 5 hours, but lividity with bluish-purplish-red discoloration is very evident by 5 to 6 hours. The discoloration remains after compression by about 12 hours and, as red cells break down, a marbling discoloration occurs, and Tardieu spots (tiny dark spots) result from capillary rupture. When lividity occurs, the rest of the body takes on a grey hue. The color of the lividity may vary depending on the cause of death, and the face is often deep reddish-purple in those with cardiac-related death. While liver mortis is occurring, the body also goes through rigor mortis, muscle contracture and stiffening, and algor mortis, cooling of the body to ambient temperature.

RIGOR MORTIS

Immediately after death, the body tends to be flaccid. However, changes occur within a few hours. **Rigor mortis** is an exaggerated contraction of muscles that occurs 2 to 6 hours after death when stores of **adenosine phosphate (ATP)**, which is necessary for muscle relaxation, are depleted. Rigor mortis is progressive, beginning with the internal organs and progressing to small muscles in the head and neck (such as the eyelids) and on to larger muscles in the trunk and extremities. Rigor mortis may be more pronounced in those with large muscles while those who are thin and frail may have less rigor mortis. Ambient temperatures may affect the onset and duration of rigor mortis with high temperatures speeding and low temperatures slowing the changes. Chemical activity usually peaks at about 12 hours and ends by 18 hours after this peak but may persist up to another 48 or more hours, at which points the muscles relax.

ALGOR MORTIS

Normal body temperature is about 37 °C, but when body functions cease at death, **algor mortis** ("cold death"), a gradual decrease in body temperature, begins within approximately one hour, and the body starts to cool by about 1 °C every hour until it reaches **ambient temperature**. The exterior surface temperature cools more rapidly than the internal temperature, and the overall rate of cooling may vary depending on the patient's internal temperature at the time of death, the

86

ambient temperature of the environment, the patient's size (muscle mass, fat), and the presence and thickness of clothing or blankets. High temperatures (internal or external) slow the cooling process. As the body cools, the skin loses elasticity and takes on a waxy appearance. This stage of the process of death ends when the temperature begins to rise again as part of **decomposition**, generally within 24 hours.

DEATH VIGIL

A death vigil entails staying with a dying person and ensuring that the person is never left alone. In some cases, the death vigil may be over within hours, but other patients may die slowly over a number of days, and family members can become exhausted, so they should be encouraged to take turns sitting vigil or to take periodic rest periods. In some cultures, a death vigil means a large number of people are present, but in other cases only one or two close family members. In either case, the nurse can support this practice by helping to make the room comfortable with adequate seating and encouraging friends/family to maintain a quiet and peaceful environment (low lights, soft music, limited conversation, and distractions). The nurse should assist with any cultural traditions that the family desires and ask the family if they want a visit from a spiritual leader/advisor (such as a priest or shaman) and help with arrangements.

POSTMORTEM CARE

The body should be prepared in order to provide a clean, peaceful impression for those family members who desire an opportunity to say good-bye before transport to a funeral home. Kindly caring for the body shows respect to the family, the continued value of the deceased, as well as modeling grief-facilitating behaviors for others present. Religious or other rituals the family may find comforting should be encouraged, as well as inviting them to participate in the preparation of the body. Explain the process and what to expect as care is given. Unless otherwise indicated by protocol or the need for autopsy, any tubes, drains, and other medical devices should be removed. Bandages should be applied, as fluids may still be expressed. A waterproof pad or incontinence brief underneath the body is helpful for containing fluids. Packing of the vagina or rectum is unnecessary. Wash the body and comb the hair. Consider dressing the body in something normalizing. It should be noted that the body may "sigh" as it is rolled and the lungs are compressed. If the area is kept cool, the decomposition process will be slowed allowing the family time to grieve.

PROVIDING SUPPORT WHEN NOTIFYING FAMILY AND COWORKERS AT TIME-OF-DEATH

The nurse should prepare to notify family and coworkers near and at the time of death by asking family members **before death is imminent** who should be notified in the event the patient's condition worsens and how that notification should be carried out (telephone, text) and should post this information prominently in the patient's **chart**. Because of HIPAA regulations regarding privacy and confidentiality, only those coworkers and friends that the patient and/or family have indicated should be notified can be contacted. (Health information remains protected under HIPAA for 50 years after a patient's death). If calling to notify a person of a death, the nurse should prepare the person first: "I'm sorry to say that I have some bad news." Then, the nurse should briefly explain that the patient has died, avoiding euphemisms, which may be misunderstood and should answer any questions the person may have. The nurse should express sympathy, "I'm so sorry for your loss," but avoid clichés such as, "He is in a better place."

PROVIDING INFORMATION AND ASSISTANCE REGARDING FUNERAL PRACTICES/PREPARATION

Some patients or family will have made **advance arrangements** for care of the body after death (cremation, burial) and funeral or memorial service, but others may be **unprepared**, so the nurse should question the family when death is imminent about whether they have made plans or the patient has expressed a preference or if there are any traditional, religious, or cultural practices that they want to carry out and need assistance with before or after the patient's death. The nurse should provide lists of local funeral homes and cremation services that are available (with price ranges if available) so that the family can more easily make decisions but should avoid making specific recommendations. If for some reason an autopsy will be scheduled, the family should be advised of when that will take place and how they can claim the body.

DEATH PRONOUNCEMENT

The death pronouncement itself is fairly straightforward, but it can be complicated by the presence of family members or friends, so the nurse must remain sensitive to their needs and emotions. Protocols for **death pronouncement** may vary somewhat but generally include:

- Gather information from medical health record and staff members if not present at the time of death
- Identify the patient, verifying patient's ID number
- Description of the body's appearance and location
- Verbal and tactile stimulation utilized and lack of response
- Check of pupillary reflex and finding of fixed and dilated pupils
- Assessment of respiratory status and lack of breathing/lung sounds
- Assessment of cardiac status and lack of pulse noted on palpation and auscultation of apical pulse for at least 60 seconds
- Note and record the official time of death
- Note family and physician notifications
- File report to CDC for those conditions that require notification if part of responsibility
- Describe notification of appropriate authorities for suspicious death or when regulations require notification of the medical examiner

DOCUMENTATION NEEDED AT THE TIME OF DEATH

Documentation needed at the time of death includes:

- Deceased name, birthdate, address, and unique patient number
- Date and time of documentation
- Reason for attending to the deceased
- List of those present at time of death
- Description of circumstances, including location and complications or disease processes that may have contributed to death
- Outline of death confirmation according to established protocol
- Outcome of assessment and time of death
- Interactions with others present, including staff members and family members
- Specific notifications, such as of spouse, children, or physician
- Description of any special requests or concerns, such as cultural practices
- Discussion regarding organ donation and plans
- Plans for disposition of body (funeral home, autopsy, body/organ donation)
- Notification of medical examiner if required by circumstances and/or regulations and reasons
- Signature, including full name, role, any professional number, and contact information (telephone)

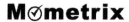

APPROPRIATE CLOSURE ACTIVITIES

When a patient has died, the nurse should utilize closure activities rather than abruptly ending association with the family, who may have developed a close relationship with the nurse. **Closure activities** may include:

- **Make a home visit**: This may be especially comforting to the family of a deceased patient and gives the family members a chance to express their feelings and ask any questions they might have and the nurse to help them cope with grief and provide information about resources, such as grief support groups, that may benefit them. The nurse should call in advance and schedule the meeting at the family's convenience and should, if they decline, respect their decision.
- **Telephone**: The nurse should call within a few days of death and a week or two later to talk with family members about how they are doing and to see if they have any questions or needs the nurse can assist with.
- **Send a card of condolence**: A card and a note about the patient and some specific memory can provide a tangible item of comfort for the family members. A card remembering the patient's birthday and at intervals, such as 3, 6, 12, and 24 months after death, is comforting to family.

Cancer Treatment and Supportive Care

Clinical Trials and Research Studies

RESEARCH PROTOCOLS FOR CANCER

A research protocol is the blueprint of a clinical trial or research study for the treatment of cancer. The National Cancer Institute defines a **research protocol** as "a detailed plan of a scientific or medical experiment, treatment, or procedure." Research protocols include a description of the study, the duration of the study, how the study will be executed, and why it is being done. The protocol will explain how many participants will be in the study, eligibility criteria for the study (including inclusion and exclusion criteria), any medications or other interventions that will be given during the course of the study (including testing), the frequency of the intervention, and how the data gathered throughout the study will be collected. Nursing staff caring for the oncology patient have a critical role in the orchestration of the research protocol. It is vitally important that the protocol be followed thoroughly and accurately to ensure the patient has the greatest chance of the intervention(s) being successful in the cancer treatment.

ELEMENTS OF A CLINICAL TRIAL PROTOCOL

Clinical trials follow a **clinical trial protocol** that has been developed by the company or sponsoring agency. All protocols should contain certain elements that define how the trial is to be performed. The protocol states the therapeutic formulation and its background plus justification for the trial and its objectives. It outlines the design of the trial in terms of patient selection and randomization, procedures for evaluating the patient at all trial stages (before, during, and after treatment), identification of study endpoints, documentation of critical adverse effects, and criteria for termination of participation. The protocol should also address data issues like statistical evaluation and publication rights. It should include information about central review procedures as well as other regulatory or administrative issues. References, other information, and model informed consent forms are usually included in the protocol as well.

NATIONAL CANCER INSTITUTE-SPONSORED CLINICAL TRIALS

A **clinical trial** is a scientifically controlled study of the safety and efficacy of a therapeutic agent (or a medical device or unique procedure) utilizing human subjects who have given informed consent in order to participate. The National Cancer Institute (NCI) at least partially oversees and funds many of these clinical trials, usually in collaboration with pharmaceutical or biotechnology companies. The NCI directly funds a number of cooperative groups that primarily monitor clinical trials, such as the Southwest Oncology Group. In order to facilitate patient selection and speed up the clinical trials process, the NCI also has set up two major programs. The first is the Cancer Trials Support Unit or CTSU, which is a centralized regulatory catalog. The CTSU lists available trials for clinical investigators and helps draw appropriate patients into the trial. The NCI has also set up a central institutional review board (CIRB), which reviews any Cooperative Group or other phase III study and makes recommendations to the local institutional review board (LIRB) where generally the head can approve changes without a meeting of the whole LIRB.

BIOPHARMACEUTICAL INDUSTRY-SPONSORED CLINICAL TRIALS

Pharmaceutical and biotechnology companies are focused on obtaining eventual approval by the Federal Drug Administration (FDA) to market the therapeutic agents being studied. Therefore, they tend to restrict the types of investigators used to conduct the clinical trials, particularly in the initial phases I and II, to allow for closer monitoring. Phase I might be confined to a single

90

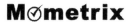

investigator and phase II might be performed in-house or by an outside concept leader. The trial design is maximized to facilitate approval by the FDA as well as the regulatory organizations in other countries where marketing is sought. The company either directly develops and manufactures or has an agreement to distribute the agent. Many of the clinical trials functions are performed by in-house personnel or hired out to contract research organizations (CROs).

PHASES OF CLINICAL TRIALS

There are four possible phases of clinical trials:

- **Phase I trials** are designed merely to test the safety of the agent in terms of maximum tolerated dose, effective administration protocol, and possible toxicities. Generally, any patient who is stable and not terminal can participate in a phase I trial.
- **Phase II trials** look at the efficacy of the agent in terms of whether it can produce a favorable response in patients with particular tumor types, using the parameters established in phase I. Patients with measurable disease but without other good treatment options are generally selected. Individuals chosen for phase I or II trials may have been treated previously for their cancer.
- **Phase III** compares the efficacy of the new agent or therapeutic protocol to the current standard in patients with measurable disease who have not been pretreated; these trials are larger and usually randomized. If the clinical trial indicates improvement over current standards, FDA approval is sought and the formulation marketed.
- **Phase IV** or postmarketing studies are done later to either promote further knowledge about the agent, including morbidity and mortality statistics, or to look at different patient populations.

INFORMED CONSENT FOR CLINICAL TRIALS

Whenever a patient undergoes a medical procedure such as surgery, written **informed consent** must be obtained. This entails thoroughly explaining the benefits, burdens, expected outcomes, and other consequences of participation to the individual. In the case of clinical trials, informed consent is vital. A patient to be enrolled in a clinical trial must be given thorough information about the study before obtaining informed consent, including information regarding the purpose, length, benefits, risks, and the costs involved. Patients are also advised regarding alternative options to participation. Only then should the patient or the patient's representative (such as a parent of an underage child) sign the informed consent document. Nurses are usually the primary clinician involved in educating the patient and obtaining informed consent. Care should be taken to avoid conflicts of interest and to recruit patients for the trial of varying race, gender, and economic background.

RESPONSIBILITIES OF NURSES INVOLVED IN RESEARCH

Nurses can serve various and often overlapping roles during the conduct of clinical trials. A research or clinical trial nurse may be employed to coordinate all aspects of the trial. Advanced practice nurses are often hired in this role. There is often a data manager or clinical research associate, who may be a nurse but is often a separately trained individual, who collects and systematizes all of the study data. Protocol treatment nurses actually administer the treatment, record responses or adverse effects, and serve to educate the patient. The team might also have a nurse researcher who does companion studies attendant to the primary investigation.

EVIDENCE-BASED GUIDELINES STEPS

Steps to evidence-based practice guidelines include:

- **Focus on the topic/methodology**: This includes outlining possible interventions/treatments for review, choosing patient populations and settings, and determining significant outcomes. Search boundaries (such as types of journals, types of studies, dates of studies) should be determined.
- **Evidence review**: This includes review of literature, critical analysis of studies, and summarizing of results, including pooled meta-analysis.
- **Expert judgment**: Recommendations based on personal experience from a number of experts may be utilized, especially if there is inadequate evidence based on review, but this subjective evidence should be explicitly acknowledged.
- **Policy considerations**: This includes cost-effectiveness, access to care, insurance coverage, availability of qualified staff, and legal implications.
- **Policy**: A written policy must be complete with recommendations. Common practice is to utilize letter guidelines, with A being the most highly recommended, usually based on the quality of supporting evidence.
- **Review**: The completed policy should be submitted to peers for review and comments before instituting the policy.

OUTCOMES EVALUATION AND EVIDENCE-BASED PRACTICE

Outcomes evaluation is an important component of evidence-based practice, which involves both internal and external research. All treatments are subjected to review to determine if they produce positive outcomes, and policies and protocols for outcomes evaluation should be in place. Outcomes evaluation includes the following:

- **Monitoring** over the course of treatment involves careful observation and record keeping that notes progress, with supporting laboratory and radiographic evidence as indicated by condition and treatment.
- **Evaluating** results includes reviewing records as well as current research to determine if outcomes are within acceptable parameters.
- **Sustaining** involves continuing the treatment while continuing to monitor and evaluate.
- **Improving** means to continue the treatment but with additions or modifications in order to improve outcomes.
- **Replacing** the treatment with a different treatment must be done if outcomes evaluation indicates that current treatment is ineffective.

Chemotherapy

PATIENT CRITERIA FOR CHEMOTHERAPEUTIC PROTOCOLS

Before administering chemotherapy or selecting an appropriate protocol, several **patient criteria** should be considered. Patients are usually given a performance score based on one of two scales: Karnofsky or Zubrod. In each, if the patient is symptomatic and either bedridden or in bed at least half of the day, they are considered poor candidates for chemotherapy. The physiological age of the individual and the possible level of toxicity versus benefit are also of primary consideration. History of prior failure of a specific chemotherapeutic regimen generally precludes its subsequent use. If the patient has diminished bone marrow, renal, hepatic, and sometimes cardiac or pulmonary function, some drugs cannot be administered. Similarly, if the patient has concomitant illnesses, the choice of drugs may be affected. Further, the patient must be able to either ingest sufficient calories during treatment or take infused nutritional support. Obese patients are often problematic because it is more difficult to determine correct dosages. Lastly, certain metabolic deficiencies must be taken into account.

CLASSIFICATION OF RESPONSE TO CHEMOTHERAPY

Patient response to a chemotherapeutic regimen is generally classified as follows:

- **Complete response**: A four-week period during which no quantifiable measurement of disease can be observed and no other lesions appear.
- **Partial response**: A four-week period during which the diameter of the primary tumor is reduced at least 50% and there are no new lesions or enlargement of previous ones; for hepatic cancers, a 30% reduction is considered a partial response.
- **Stable disease**: Either some reduction or no more than 25% increase in tumor diameter within an eight-week period and no new tumor sites.
- **Relapse or progression**: More than 25% increase above either pre-treatment tumor size or dimension after optimal regression, or metastasis to other areas.

The size of the tumor is generally measured as the aggregate of all tumor masses. Protocols are generally continued for a few cycles with positive responses, changed with negative ones, and reevaluated with stable disease.

ROLE OF CHEMOTHERAPY IN MANAGEMENT OF ADVANCED AND METASTATIC CANCER

When chemotherapeutic agents are used to treat **advanced or metastatic disease**, their effectiveness can be measured in many ways. In general, the possible results from the use of chemotherapeutic agents can include: a complete response with no evidence of disease after a certain time period, a partial response with at least 50% reduction in tumor burden, or a simple alleviation of symptoms and improvement in quality of life. In the case of metastatic cancer spread, chemotherapy is really the only method of treatment. Solid tumors have rarely been cured (i.e., evidencing a complete response) by chemotherapy except in cases of germ cell cancer of the testis. A number of primarily lymphoid-derived cancers, however, have been successfully treated with chemotherapy. These include acute lymphoid leukemia, Hodgkin's disease, and gestational choriocarcinoma. Ovarian cancer, small cell lung cancer, and acute myeloid leukemia have been obliterated in some instances by the use of chemotherapy.

RELATION OF CELL CYCLE, CELL-CYCLE TIME, GROWTH FRACTION OF TUMOR, AND TUMOR BURDEN TO CHEMOTHERAPY TREATMENT

- **Cell cycle** is the action of cell reproduction. This occurs in all cells, including cancer cells. Certain cancer treatments can be targeted to affect cancer cells at specific points within the reproductive cycle.
- **Cell-cycle time** is the length of time required for a cell to complete an entire reproductive cycle. This is important in formulating cancer treatments because some cancer cells will have a longer cell-cycle time than others. This can affect the length of time the cell spends in each phase of the reproductive cycle.
- **Growth fraction of tumor** is the number of cancer cells that are going through the reproductive cycle. This is measured in a percent. The percentage of dividing cells at any time is important for treatments that target specific phases of the reproductive cycle.
- **Tumor burden** is the size of a tumor measured in the number of cells that comprise it. This helps to determine the difficulty in treating a cancer because the smaller the tumor, the more responsive it will be to treatment.

MAJOR CLASSIFICATIONS OF CHEMOTHERAPY DRUGS

Chemotherapeutic agents are classified as to how they work in conjunction with the various phases of the cell cycle. They are known as either **cell cycle specific**, meaning they work at a particular phase of the cell cycle, or as **cell cycle nonspecific**, meaning they are active throughout all phases of the cell cycle. Chemotherapeutic agents can be further classified into the following major categories: alkylating agents, anti-metabolites, anthracyclines, anti-tumor antibiotics, camptothecins, epothilones, vinca alkaloids, taxanes, and platinums. Anti-metabolites are active in the "S" phase of the cell cycle and are considered cell cycle specific. Epothilones, taxanes, and vinca alkaloids are specific to the "M" phase of the cell cycle. These agents are also known as mitotic inhibitors. Alkylating agents, anthracyclines, and platinums are all considered cell cycle nonspecific agents.

CELL CYCLE NONSPECIFIC CLASSES OF CHEMOTHERAPY DRUGS

The cell cycle is composed of **four phases**: G1, S1, G2, and M. Many chemotherapeutic agents are active in the "S" phase of the cell cycle in which DNA replication is most active. Chemotherapeutic agents that work in all phases of the cell cycle and are not specific to one particular phase are known as **cell cycle phase nonspecific agents**. The **alkylating agents** work by directly damaging cell DNA to prevent the cancer cell from reproducing. Alkylating agents work in all phases of the cell cycle and are most active in the resting phase of the cell cycle. Examples of alkylating agents include nitrogen mustard, carmustine, lomustine, busulfan, thiotepa, and cyclophosphamide. The **platinum class** of chemotherapeutic agents are also cell cycle phase nonspecific. These agents work by inhibiting DNA synthesis, transcription, and function by cross-linking DNA subunits. Agents in the platinum class include cisplatin, carboplatin, and oxaliplatin.

ALKYLATING AGENTS

The alkylating agents are the oldest class of chemotherapy drugs. They work by interfering with the cell's DNA and inhibiting cell growth. Because of the way these agents interfere with a cell's DNA, there is a risk of long-term damage to the **bone marrow** and subsequently the development of **leukemia**. The risk of leukemia development is at its highest 5-10 years post treatment and is also increased with higher doses administered. Alkylating agents include the nitrogen mustards, nitrosoureas (including carmustine and streptozocin), alkyl sulfonates (including busulfan), triazines (including dacarbazine), and the ethyleneamines. The alkylating agents are used in the treatment of leukemia, lymphoma (including Hodgkin lymphoma), multiple myeloma, sarcoma, lung, breast, brain, and ovarian cancers.

- **Dacarbazine (DTIC)** is an alkylating agent used in the treatment of melanoma, Hodgkin lymphoma, sarcoma, and neuroblastoma.
- **Carmustine (BCNU)** is an alkylating agent used to treat primary brain tumors, Hodgkin lymphoma, melanoma, and lung and colon cancer.
- **Carboplatin** is an alkylating agent used in the treatment of ovarian, lung, head and neck, endometrial, bladder, breast, and cervical cancers. It is also used in the treatment of central nervous system tumors and sarcomas. It can be administered intravenously and also given as an intraperitoneal infusion for the treatment of ovarian cancer.
- **Cisplatin** is the sister agent of Carboplatin. It is an alkylating agent used in the treatment of testicular, ovarian, bladder, head and neck, esophageal, lung, breast, cervical, stomach, and prostate cancers. It is also used in the treatment of lymphomas, multiple myeloma, neuroblastomas, melanoma, and mesothelioma. Cisplatin is considered an irritant agent. It can be administered intravenously or as an intraperitoneal infusion.

Nitrosoureas are a type of alkylating agent that are not cell cycle dependent. Nitrosoureas add alkyl groups to DNA as do other alkylating agents. Examples include carmustine (BCNU), which is approved for use with brain tumors and various lymphoid cancers and streptozocin (Zanosar), which is primarily used to treat metastatic islet cell carcinoma.

ANTI-TUMOR ANTIBIOTICS

Anti-tumor antibiotics are cell cycle nonspecific agents that act during multiple phases of the cell cycle. Anti-tumor antibiotics are derived from byproducts of the species of soil fungus *Streptomyces*. They work by binding with DNA to prevent the synthesis of RNA. They also prohibit cell growth by preventing DNA replication. Anthracyclines, chromomycins, and a few miscellaneous chemotherapeutic agents make up the anti-tumor antibiotic class. Doxorubicin, daunorubicin, epirubicin, mitoxantrone, idarubicin, dactinomycin, plicamycin, mitomycin, and bleomycin are examples of anti-tumor antibiotics. Common side effects with anti-tumor antibiotics include neutropenia, thrombocytopenia, alopecia, fever, headache, nausea and vomiting, anorexia, peripheral neuropathy, cardiac toxicity (with anthracyclines), pulmonary toxicity (with bleomycin), skin rash, photosensitivity, and changes in urine color (with mitomycin). Lifetime dose limitations of the anthracyclines are recommended due to the risk of permanent cardiac damage. Anti-tumor antibiotics are used in the treatment of leukemias, lymphomas, and solid tumor cancers.

COMMON ANTI-TUMOR ANTIBIOTICS MEDICATIONS

Anti-tumor antibiotics act by interfering with DNA in some manner. Commonly used agents include the following:

- **Bleomycin (Blenoxane)**: Induces DNA strand breaks and is used to treat Hodgkin's and non-Hodgkin's lymphoma, head and neck squamous cell carcinomas, reproductive system cancers and others
- **Dactinomycin (Cosmegen)**: Interacts with DNA to prohibit transcription and is used to treat some unique cancers, such as Wilms' tumor, Ewing's and other sarcomas, connective tissue-derived tumors and more
- **Daunorubicin (Cerubidine)**: Intercalating agent that is approved for use with acute myeloid and lymphocytic leukemia
- **Doxorubicin hydrochloride (Adriamycin)**: Intercalating agent and is used for leukemias and lymphomas as well as several solid tumors and multiple myeloma
- **Doxorubicin, liposome (Doxil)**: Liposome preparation of intercalating agent and is used primarily for Kaposi's sarcoma and metastatic ovarian cancer
- **Mitomycin C (Mutamycin)**: Inhibitor of both RNA and DNA synthesis that is approved for Aden carcinomas of the pancreas and stomach, and also used for other cancers
- **Mitoxantrone (Novantrone)**: Anthracycline, approved for AML and prostate cancer but also included in treatments for breast and hepatocellular carcinomas and lymphomas.
- **Plicamycin (Mithracin)**: Primarily used to lower malignancy-induced spikes in calcium levels.

CELL CYCLE SPECIFIC CLASSES OF CHEMOTHERAPY DRUGS
ANTI-METABOLITES

Anti-metabolites were among the first chemotherapeutic agents noted to be effective in treating cancer. They are **cell cycle specific**, attacking at specific phases of the cell cycle. Anti-metabolites work by interfering with specific substances within the cell, thereby impairing their ability to divide. The anti-metabolites are further classified by the substances in which they interfere. Anti-metabolites are used in the treatment of leukemia, breast, ovarian, and GI cancers. Examples of anti-metabolites include methotrexate (a folic acid antagonist), 5-FU, cytarabine, capecitabine, gemcitabine (pyrimidine antagonists), 6-mercaptopurine (a purine antagonist), and cladribine and fludarabine (adenosine deaminase inhibitors).

- **5-FU** is an anti-metabolite used in the treatment of colon, rectal, breast, GI, head and neck, and ovarian cancers.
- **Cytarabine** is an anti-metabolite used in the treatment of leukemia and lymphoma. It can be administered intravenously, intramuscularly, or subcutaneously. Cytarabine is one of only a few chemotherapeutic agents that can be administered intrathecally, for direct administration into the cerebral spinal fluid.
- **Capecitabine** is an anti-metabolite used in the treatment of breast and colorectal cancers.
- **Fludarabine** is used to treat chronic leukemia and non-Hodgkin lymphoma.

MITOTIC INHIBITORS

Mitotic inhibitors include the plant alkaloids and taxanes as well as the epothilones. They work by **stopping mitosis** and are **cell cycle specific**, working in the "M" phase of the cell cycle. With the arrest of mitosis and inhibition of necessary enzymes, the proteins needed for cellular reproduction are not made. Mitotic inhibitors are used in the treatment of breast and lung cancers, as well as in the treatment of myeloma, lymphoma, and leukemia. Paclitaxel is a plant alkaloid and taxane that is used in the treatment of breast, ovarian, lung, bladder, prostate, melanoma, and esophageal cancer. Ixabepilone is used in the treatment of metastatic or locally advanced breast cancer. Vinblastine is a plant alkaloid used in the treatment of testicular, breast, lung, head and neck, and bladder cancer. It is also used in the treatment of sarcoma, lymphoma, and choriocarcinoma.

VINCA ALKALOIDS

Vinca alkaloids **inhibit tubulin polymerization** during the G_2 phase of the cell cycle, preventing mitosis and cell division. At present, there are three available drugs in this category: Vinblastine (Velban, etc.), vincristine (Oncovin), and vinorelbine (Navelbine). The first two are primarily used to treat hematologic- or lymphoid-derived cancers such as Hodgkin's disease. Vinblastine is effective for the treatment of solid tumors as well. Vincristine is used to treat some unique tumors, such as Wilms' tumor and neuroblastoma. Vinorelbine is approved for use in cases of metastatic breast cancer and non-small cell lung cancer.

TAXANES

Taxanes usually act by **inhibiting the mitotic spindle apparatus** through stabilization of tubulin polymers; this mechanism ultimately leads to cell death during mitosis. The most commonly used taxanes are docetaxel (Taxotere) and paclitaxel (Taxol). Docetaxel is sanctioned by the FDA for metastatic breast carcinoma and non-small cell lung cancer, but is also used for other epithelial-derived neoplasms, stomach cancers, and head and neck cancers. Paclitaxel (Taxol) is administered intravenously and is classified as an irritant agent. It is used in the treatment of breast, ovarian, lung, prostate, and esophageal cancers, as well as melanoma.

TOPOISOMERASE INHIBITORS

Topoisomerase inhibitors are substances that block the action of the topoisomerase enzymes. **Topoisomerase enzymes** are substances that break and rejoin DNA strands that are needed for cells to divide and grow. Blocking of these enzymes then leads to cellular death of the cancer cells. Topoisomerase inhibitors are divided into topoisomerase I and topoisomerase II. Camptothecin and its derivatives (including irinotecan) are examples of **topoisomerase I inhibitors**. Doxorubicin, etoposide, and mitoxantrone are examples of **topoisomerase II inhibitors**. Irinotecan is a plant alkaloid and topoisomerase I inhibitor used in the treatment of metastatic colon or rectal cancer. Etoposide is a plant alkaloid and topoisomerase II inhibitor used in the treatment of testicular, bladder, prostate, lung, stomach, uterine, and brain cancers. It is also indicated for the treatment of some lymphomas, sarcomas, and neuroblastoma. Mitoxantrone is an anti-tumor antibiotic and topoisomerase II inhibitor used in the treatment of prostate and breast cancer, as well as leukemia and lymphoma.

UNIQUE CHEMOTHERAPEUTIC AGENTS

There are a few agents used in chemotherapeutic protocols **that have unique structures and modes of action**. Among these is gallium nitrate (Ganite), a heavy metal that inhibits iron metabolism (and thereby limits tumor growth) and also suppresses blood calcium levels, which are often elevated in the presence of malignancies. Platinating agents, such as oxaliplatin (Eloxatin), that induce apoptosis by inserting platinum to break DNA strands have been used to treat metastatic colorectal cancer. Several cryoprotectant agents, such as amifostine (Ethyol), act as free-radical scavengers. Other drugs include various forms of asparaginase, which cleaves the essential amino acid asparagine.

ADJUVANT AND NEOADJUVANT CHEMOTHERAPY

Both adjuvant and neoadjuvant chemotherapy involve the use of various drugs and chemicals to control the spread of disease, in this case the metastatic spread of cancer. The difference between the two centers around the time frame in which they are administered. Adjuvant chemotherapy is given after apparent obliteration of the primary tumor by surgery or radiation in order to reduce the possibility of metastasis. Its effectiveness is gauged in terms of relapse-free survival time or the overall survival rate. Neoadjuvant chemotherapy is the use of agents to lower tumor burden before treatment of the primary cancer by radiation or surgery. Distant micrometastases as well as the bulk of the primary tumor can be shrunk by this approach, and it can possibly lead to more conservative removal tactics. Neoadjuvant chemotherapy has been effective in treating a number of cancers in terms of preservation of the affected organ and its function.

COMBINATION OR CYCLIC CHEMOTHERAPY

Combination chemotherapy is the use of more than one form of chemotherapy for the reduction of tumor load. The rationale is that each individual can potentially be resistant to a particular drug or become resistant to a particular drug during treatment, while theoretically still responding to other agents. Therefore, chemotherapeutic agents selected for combination protocols should: 1) have demonstrated disease-specific anti-tumor activity, 2) have different modes of action, and 3) be given under optimal dosage and timing conditions. An additional consideration is the time it takes the surrounding normal tissue to recover from the toxicity caused by the agent, which generally means that the drug should be given for as short a time as therapeutically possible. One approach is to use **cyclic chemotherapy** in which different drug combinations are given in cycles. Usually, two different combinations are administered in alternating cycles, but some protocols have used all of the desired reagents at unique times or concentrations in a particular cycle. To date, the efficacy of cyclic chemotherapy regimens has only been demonstrated in hematological tumors and a few solid tumors.

NOVEL APPROACHES TO CHEMOTHERAPY

Many newer, more novel approaches to chemotherapy are either in development or have limited years of study. The effectiveness of some of these types of drugs is only transitory. Commercially available retinoid (Vitamin A) derivatives like isotretinoin (Accutane) fall into this category as do compounds similar to Vitamin D, cyclo-oxygenase inhibitors, and hypomethylating compounds. Drugs that can prevent angiogenesis or new vascularization required for tumor growth are promising in theory but as yet remain unproven. Agents that can inhibit signal transduction pathways, such as epithelial growth factors, also offer promise. Gene therapy has been performed in animal models but it is only at the clinical trial stage for humans, at present. Cancer vaccines incorporating human tumor antigens are also being studied.

EMERGING METHODS FOR IDENTIFICATION OF POSSIBLE NEW CHEMOTHERAPEUTIC AGENTS

Computer modeling is currently being utilized for what is known as mechanistic drug development. This process uses computer analysis to calculate the chemical constitution of promising new drug formulations. Another technique is **combinatorial chemistry**. In this approach the binding capacity of a compound is tested against known targets coupled to a solid phase. Those substances that bind well are examined functionally for further potential utility. Computer analysis of tumor cells is also being used to hunt for either genes or gene expressions using genomics, or protein sections using proteomics. Using these methodologies, potential future therapeutic targets can be identified.

Biotherapy and Hormonal Therapy

TYPES OF BIOLOGICAL AND MOLECULAR TREATMENTS

Types of biological and molecular treatments used to treat cancer include the following:

1. **Cytokines** make up the largest group of biotherapy agents. They are proteins that are produced by immune cells that interfere with the normal actions of a cell. Examples include interferon, interleukins, tumor necrosis factor, and blood growth factors.
2. **Monoclonal antibodies** recognize specific antigens on the outside of cancer cells and trigger an immune response targeted at these cells.
3. **Fusion proteins** function to cause destruction of cancer cells.
4. **Effector cells** are specialized immune cells that are taken from the patient and then given by IV infusion.
5. **Immunomodulators** are less specific than some other biotherapy agents, but function to trigger an immune response.
6. **Retinoids** are produced by vitamin A and function in cell growth and function.
7. **Vaccines** introduce the body's immune system to a specific antigen in order to form antibodies against the foreign agent.
8. **Molecular targeted therapies** are comprised of various agents that interfere with normal function of cancer cells.
9. **Gene therapy** is still considered an experimental treatment. Its goal is to directly interfere with a cancer cell in order to destroy it.

> **Review Video: Immunomodulators and Immunosuppressors**
> Visit mometrix.com/academy and enter code: 666131

BIOTHERAPY

Biotherapy is a form of treatment that is created from natural components. Biotherapy treatments may be capable of changing the way the human body reacts to cancer cells. Most biotherapy agents are formed from **cytokines** which trigger the immune system to attack malignant cells. These agents are used to interrupt normal cell functions that occur within malignant cells. They can interfere with cell growth and disrupt the production of necessary proteins and enzymes by the cancer cells.

Examples of biotherapy include specialized **antibodies and vaccines**. These antibodies are not only used to treat cancer, though. Because they target cancer cells, they may also be used for diagnosing and staging cancer. Radioactive material can be attached to the antibodies, and scans can be performed to detect the areas of antibody distribution. This can identify specific areas of the body that are affected by cancer and determine how advanced the disease may have become.

CLASSIFICATIONS, PURPOSE, AND RISK FACTORS OF INTERFERON

Interferons are a naturally occurring protein found in the body. When used in medicine, interferon belongs to the classification cytokines, and their function is to change the response of the cells of the immune system, thereby slowing the growth of cancer cells. There are three classifications of interferons: alpha, beta, and gamma. Interferons can increase the effectiveness of the medication zidovudine, which increases risk of toxicity. Interferon can interfere with excretion of theophylline, so levels should be closely monitored. The most common interferon used to treat cancer is interferon alpha. Used to treat a variety of cancers, interferon alpha-2B has a black box warning for potentially causing neurological, psychiatric, immune/autoimmune, and ischemic emergencies that can be fatal. It can cause hepatotoxicity as well as hypertriglyceridemia. If severe hypertriglyceridemia (triglyceride levels of 500 mg/dL or higher) persists, treatment with interferon should be discontinued. Other side effects of interferon alpha-2B include flu-like symptoms such as fever, myalgia, and fatigue. Interferon can also cause neutropenia, anemia, and thrombocytopenia. Hematologic effects should be monitored and dosages adjusted or held according to severity.

MONOCLONAL ANTIBODIES

Monoclonal antibodies (mAbs) can be divided into two types: unconjugated and conjugated.

- **Unconjugated monoclonal antibodies** are those not bound to a drug, toxin, or radioactive substance. Unconjugated mAbs may also be referred to as naked mAbs and are the most commonly used monoclonal antibodies. Trastuzumab is an example of an unconjugated mAb, commonly used to treat breast and endometrial cancers.
- **Conjugated mAbs** are joined to radioactive isotopes, chemotherapeutic agents, or toxins to poison the cancer cells they are targeting. Conjugated mAbs work by transporting the associated anticancer agents directly to the cancer cells. Conjugated mAbs do not attach to hormones.
  - Ibritumomab is indicated in combination with rituximab in the treatment of relapsed or refractory low-grade, follicular, or transformed B-cell NHL.
  - Gemtuzumab is indicated for the treatment of CD33 positive acute myeloid leukemia.
  - Iodine-131 tositumomab is indicated for the treatment of CD20 positive, follicular NHL (not used in combination with rituximab).
  - Alemtuzumab is indicated for the treatment of B-cell chronic lymphocytic leukemia.
  - Ipilimumab is for the treatment of unresectable or metastatic melanoma, metastatic colon cancer, and hepatocellular carcinoma, amongst others. Hypersensitivity to ipilimumab can result in severe and fatal immune-mediated adverse reactions as a result of T-cell activation and proliferation; therefore, patients must be closely monitored upon initial administration. The most common manifestations of these reactions include enterocolitis, hepatitis, dermatitis, neuropathy, and endocrinopathy.

AVAILABILITY

In 2021, the FDA approved its 100th mAb for the treatment of a wide variety of types of cancer and disease including leukemia, lymphoma, breast and colorectal cancers, melanoma, neuroblastoma, multiple myeloma, non-small cell lung carcinoma, bladder cancer, and urothelial carcinoma—a list that continues to grow as research progresses.

MECHANISMS OF ACTION OF ANTITUMOR MONOCLONAL ANTIBODIES

Monoclonal antibodies (mAb) are antibodies that have been derived from a single clone or cell line. They contain unique amino acid sequences directed against specific epitopes or immunological sites on an antigen. Antitumor mAbs generally participate in tumor cell death in one of three ways. First, they are able to bind to cell-surface receptors. Next, the mAbs either impede the binding of other ligands and some functions or they can cause cross linkage between several sites. Monoclonal antibodies can induce antibody-dependent cell-mediated cytotoxicity (ADCC) in certain cancer cell types, particularly in the presence of certain cytokines such as IL-2. Here, the monoclonal antibody is specific for Fc (constant region) receptors on the target tumor cells. When the mAb binds to the tumor cell, NK (natural killer) lymphocytes and/or neutrophils are recruited to the area and cytotoxicity is induced. Complement-dependent cytotoxicity (CDC) can also be initiated in certain types of tumor cells in the presence of mAbs of certain classes, particularly IgG1. The complement cascade is composed of a group of plasma antigens that participate in tumor cell death by directly lysing the cells, promoting inflammation, and/or recruiting phagocytic leukocytes.

AVAILABLE NAKED MONOCLONAL ANTIBODIES

TREATMENT OF LYMPHOMA AND LEUKEMIA

There are three licensed monoclonal antibodies available for treatment of lymphoma and leukemia in the naked form. The first mAb is **rituximab** (Rituxan), which is a chimeric IgG1 directed against the CD20 antigen and is primarily used to treat chronic lymphocytic leukemia (CLL). Rituximab is effective because it can initiate both antibody-dependent cell-mediated and complement-dependent cytotoxicity, and it also can interrupt certain signaling pathways. Patients should be closely monitored during administration of rituximab, as it has been associated with infusion-related fatalities within 24 hours of infusion. The second mAb is **ofatumumab**, which like rituximab is another IgG1 mAb that targets the CD20 antigen to treat chronic lymphocytic leukemia. The third mAb is **alemtuzumab** (Campath), which is a humanized rat mAb class IgG1 specific for the CD52 antigen. It is sanctioned for treatment of both CLL and prolymphocytic leukemia (PLL), and it can induce both ADCC and CDC.

TRIALS TO TREAT SOLID TUMORS

The first naked monoclonal antibody available for treatment of **solid tumors** was trastuzumab, a humanized rat monoclonal of the IgG1 class directed against the HER2 antigen (a tyrosine kinase). It is used for HER2-positive breast cancer and acts through ADCC, CDC, and receptor blockage. Bevacizumab (Avastin) has also been FDA-approved after showing statistically significant results in treating metastatic solid tumors, particularly colorectal cancer. Other monoclonal antibodies approved for the treatment of metastatic colorectal cancer include cetuximab and panitumumab (both which target EGFR).

IMMUNOCONJUGATES

Immunoconjugates are compounds formed by the attachment of other molecules to antibodies. In the context of treatments for malignancies, immunoconjugates are usually monoclonal antibodies to which reagents that potentiate cell killing are attached. The most commonly utilized immunoconjugates are called radioimmunoconjugates. They have radioisotopes that emit primarily either alpha or beta particles attached to the mAb. Conjugates that have monoclonal antibodies attached to either cytokines or toxins (termed immuno-cytokines or immunotoxins, respectively) are also commonly used. Sometimes monoclonals are developed with two specificities, against both the tumor and certain ligands of interest. Other unique delivery systems include antibody-directed enzyme prodrug therapy (ADEPT) and immunoliposomes.

RADIOISOTOPES USED IN RADIOIMMUNOCONJUGATES

Radioisotopes have varying half-lives and maximum energies. They can emit alpha (α) particles, beta (β) particles, and/or gamma (γ) rays; the particles have differing ranges of emission depending upon the isotope. Isotopes that emit α particles, or helium nuclei, have a higher maximum energy and a shorter range than β-emitters, making them ideal for the control of micrometastases. They include actinium 225 (^{225}Ac), astatine 211 (^{211}At), and bismuth 213 (^{213}Bi). Beta-emitters are better choices for the treatment of bulky tumors because they have a longer range of emission. However, some β-emitters, such as iodine 131 (^{131}I) and rhenium 188 (^{188}Re) also give off γ rays, thus dictating patient segregation. Pure β-emitters include yttrium 90 (^{90}Y), copper 67 (^{67}Cu), and lutetium 177 (^{177}Lu).

RADIOIMMUNOCONJUGATES LICENSED OR UNDERGOING TRIALS FOR RADIOIMMUNOTHERAPY OF LYMPHOMAS

There are two licensed **radioimmunoconjugates** for radioimmunotherapy (RIT) of **non-Hodgkin's lymphoma**. They are: tositumomab (Bexxar) and ibritumomab (Zevalin). Both are directed against the CD20 antigen and are murine monoclonal antibodies. Bexxar is an IgG2a class antibody coupled to ^{131}I, and Zevalin is a class IgG1 monoclonal with attached ^{90}Y. Since mAbs tend to segregate in the liver or spleen, a naked anti-CD antibody is usually administered first so that when the radiolabeled antibodies are given later, they will be shunted to the tumor site. ^{177}Lu-lilotomab is currently in trials as a single-dose radioimmunoconjugate for the treatment of patients with NHL that failed immunochemotherapy or have relapsed.

RADIOIMMUNOCONJUGATES BEING STUDIED FOR RIT OF LEUKEMIAS AND SOLID TUMORS

Tagged monoclonal antibodies directed against specific lineage antigens (such as CD33, CD666 or CD25) in **leukemia** patients have been studied and appear promising. For solid tumors, the effectiveness of radioimmunotherapy is more equivocal. Many trials have used RIT for treatments of neurological tumors, such as brain tumors and metastatic neuroblastoma. At present, there are clinical trials for yttrium 90-labeled mAbs for treatment of colorectal cancer (hMN14, also called labetuzumab and CEA-Cide) directed against the carcinoembryonic antigen (CEA) and ovarian cancer (pemtumomab or Theragyn) specific for the MUC-1 antigen.

TARGETED THERAPIES

Targeted therapies are a type of cancer treatment that targets specific molecules involved in cancer cell growth and survival. **Targeted therapies** differ from traditional chemotherapy in that traditional chemotherapy acts on all rapidly dividing cells, including both normal and cancerous cells. Targeted therapies only interfere with specific molecules, thereby lessening some of the side effects commonly associated with traditional chemotherapy. They are considered **cytostatic**, meaning they focus on blocking tumor cell proliferation, as opposed to cytotoxic. A targeted therapy may be a small molecule drug or a synthetic antibody designed to attack certain targets on cancer cells. Targeted therapies act in a variety of different ways. Mechanisms of action include preventing growth signaling in the tumor cell, interfering with the development of tumor blood vessels, promoting cell death, stimulating the immune system to destroy cancer cells, and delivering toxic drugs to the cancer cells themselves. Much focus and attention have been aimed at the further advancement and development of targeted therapies for many diseases, including cancer.

EXAMPLES

Imatinib mesylate is a type of targeted therapy used to treat gastrointestinal stromal tumors and chronic leukemia. Imatinib works by inhibiting the cellular enzyme tyrosine kinase, thereby inhibiting cell growth. **Gefitinib** is another example of a targeted therapy used in cancer treatment. Gefitinib works by blocking the epidermal growth factor receptor, which is often found in higher quantities on a cancer cell. Epidermal growth factor receptors signal cells to grow and divide. When this signal is blocked, the cancer cell will cease to grow and divide. Gefitinib is used in the treatment of advanced non-small cell lung cancer.

LIMITATIONS AND SIDE EFFECTS

One of the limitations of targeted therapy is that, over time, cancer cells can become **resistant**, rendering the targeted therapy less effective or ineffective. Resistance can occur in one of two ways:

- The target can change through mutation so that the targeted therapy no longer interacts well with it.
- The tumor itself can find a new pathway for it to grow that does not depend on the target.

To combat the issue of resistance, combination therapies may be used.

Another limitation of targeted therapy is that it may be difficult to **identify** particular targets for drug development due to the target's structure or its function within the cancer cell.

Although some of the side effects associated with traditional chemotherapy may be less with the use of targeted therapies, there are still significant and substantial **side effects** associated with targeted therapies. Diarrhea, liver problems, skin problems (including acneiform rash, dry skin, nail changes, and hair depigmentation), problems with blood clotting and wound healing, hypertension, and in rare instances gastrointestinal perforation have been reported with the use of targeted therapies.

TISSUE-SPECIFIC PROMOTERS TO TARGET GENE EXPRESSION

Tissue-specific promoters are used in **gene transfer vectors** in order to turn on gene expression in cancer cells preferentially over normal cells. Genes involved in the transcription process are ideal choices. Some of these promoters are tumor-associated, meaning they have broad specificity in many types of malignant cells. These include fragments that target the specialized DNA polymerase known as telomerase, as well as the vascular endothelial growth factor system. Some promoters are particular to certain tumors. Other promoters used are inducible, which means that they are activated transiently and only under certain conditions. These inducible genes are turned on when exposed to various stresses, such as irradiation, certain drugs, heat, hypoxia, or low levels of glucose. The most prominent example is the multidrug resistance gene-1 (MDR-1), which is induced by 3 drugs in combination.

CONDITIONALLY REPLICATIVE VIRUSES FOR TARGETING GENE EXPRESSION

Conditionally replicative viruses are engineered viruses that can still replicate but are altered to either delete genes involving cell-cycle regulation or to add genetic material that promotes control of replication. Generally, the desired endpoint is lysis of the tumor cells. Adenovirus vectors are the most common example of this type of conditionally replicative virus. They have been developed for use in a variety of malignancies including hepatocellular carcinoma, prostate cancer, and estrogen-responsive breast cancer. A popular target is the E1A gene, which is essential for early viral replication.

VECTOR TARGETING

Vector targeting is the attachment to vectors of various molecules that recognize tissue or cancer-specific sites to increase their efficiency. Generally, ligands that bind to cell-specific receptors are used. Only molecules that can exist in the cellular matrix without being destroyed or neutralized are effective candidates. Adenovirus and retroviral vectors are utilized for vector targeting as well as some non-viral vectors. Bifunctional bridging agents with sites that bind to both the viral molecule and the desired cell surface molecule are often used in the viral vectors. Typically, non-viral vectors are highly positively charged, and agents that neutralize this charge (like polyethylene glycol) are used as targeting agents to prevent clumping of red blood cells. Non-viral vectors are often enclosed within liposomes to increase their transferability.

MOLECULARLY TARGETED THERAPY

Molecularly targeted therapy is any treatment modality that targets a genetically defined abnormality in a malignancy or the pathways that are induced by these genetic abnormalities. At present, these treatment modalities and their modes of action are as follows:

- **All-trans retinoic acid (ATRA)**: Restores function of retinoic acid receptors in acute promyelocytic leukemia (APL), permitting differentiation.
- **Imatinib (Gleevec)**: A tyrosine kinase inhibitor, preventing chromosomal translocations and point mutations in diseases such as chronic myeloid leukemia (CML) and gastrointestinal stromal tumor (GIST), as well as diseases linked to changes in platelet-derived growth factor receptor.
- **Oncogene inhibitors**: Includes inhibitors of mutations of FLT3 in acute myeloid leukemia (AML), and the signal transduction genes RAF and RAS. More recently, BRAF/MEK dual-inhibitors were FDA-approved in the treatment of advanced melanomas. These act on the MAPK/ERK pathway.

FACTORS INFLUENCING RESPONSE RATE

Complete responses to available molecularly targeted therapies are currently very rare. Often there is an **initial partial response with later relapse**. The success of these types of therapies depends in large part on three factors:

- First, patients need to be identified early in the course of their disease before multiple mutations have occurred, obscuring the effect of the targeted therapy.
- Second, response rates appear to be dependent on the presence of specific mutations, which need to be identified by diagnostic assays; patients with those mutations are more likely candidates for successful treatment.
- Finally, some individuals are initially resistant and others are responsive at the outset but later develop resistance; this means that all the mechanisms of potential relapse need to monitored.

AGENTS THAT TARGET CELL CYCLE AND APOPTOSIS

In theory, a variety of proteins controlling the **cell cycle** are good candidates for molecularly-targeted therapy as they undergo changes in malignancies. The cyclins and the kinases and kinase inhibitors that depend on them are of most interest, but most studies remain in the clinical trial phase. Other restriction points in the cell cycle are also potential targets, such as p53 and various transcription factors. Since apoptosis is circumvented in malignant cells, agents that induce this cell death are of great interest. In particular, molecules targeting tumor necrosis factor, the mitochondrial integrity family called BCL-2, and caspase, as well as associated ligands have been studied.

THERAPEUTIC AGENTS WITH OTHER TYPES OF MOLECULAR TARGETS

There are other types of potential targets related to malignancy development. Several of these are related to chromosomal or genetic stability. Telomerase is a type of reverse transcriptase activated primarily in tumors. It catalyzes the elongation of telomeres, which normally stabilize the chromosome. Thus, telomerase has emerged as a prime molecular target in recent trials. Molecules directed against genetic regions that are unstable and associated with high cancer rates, such as mismatch-repair and BCRA1 and 2 genes, are also candidates. Other types of agents include those targeting specific signaling proteins that act prior to known mutational sites and ones directed against markers on the cell surface of malignant cells. There are a number of therapeutic agents in the last category that are aimed at the CD20 cell-surface receptor found with B-cell cancers, such as rituximab (Rituxan) and several radiolabeled agents.

AGENTS THAT TARGET ANGIOGENESIS

Angiogenesis is the formation of new blood vessels during the process of tumor development. Agents that control angiogenesis can suppress cell growth and multiplication, but they do not actually kill cells. Nevertheless, these agents may prove promising in conjunction with other types of therapies, and several are undergoing clinical trials. Targets include mutations of genes involved in regulation of angiogenesis, such as the von Hippel-Lindau (VHL) gene and the vascular endothelial growth factor (VEGF) gene. The monoclonal antibody directed against VEGR, called bevacizumab or Avastin, has shown limited results, but further, more well-defined studies are required.

EPIDERMAL GROWTH FACTOR RECEPTOR INHIBITORS

Epidermal growth factor receptor is a protein that influences cancer growth in different types of cancers. It is found in abnormally high levels on the surface of many types of cancer cells, causing them to excessively divide in its presence. Increased EGFR is associated with more aggressive tumors, recurrence, poorer prognosis, and resistance to endocrine therapy.

EGFR inhibitors are classified as either tyrosine kinase inhibitors or monoclonal antibodies, depending on the way they are used to treat the cancer. Epidermal growth factor receptor inhibitors that are classified as monoclonal antibodies work by blocking the epidermal growth factor receptor protein present on the surface of the cancer cell that causes excessive cell division and subsequent tumor growth. EGFR inhibitors are used to treat breast, colon, pancreatic and non-small-cell cancers. Lapatinib is an epidermal growth factor receptor inhibitor used in the treatment of metastatic breast cancer. Gefitinib is an EGFR inhibitor commonly used in non-small-cell lung cancer. Because EGFR inhibitors are targeted agents, they can have less side effects than traditional chemotherapy, but cutaneous side effects are seen frequently. These include acneiform eruptions, xerosis, paronychia, and eczema.

AGENTS THAT TARGET GROWTH-STIMULATORY PATHWAYS

Agents directed against the epidermal growth factor receptor (EGFR) family target **growth-stimulatory pathways**. To date, no other group has been as well defined. These agents can be divided into two categories, depending on their target. The first category is made up of molecules that react with EGFR, which is either overexpressed intact or in a shortened form in a variety of cancers. The two main agents in this group are the small molecular weight tyrosine kinase inhibitor gefitinib (Iressa) and the monoclonal antibody trastuzumab (Herceptin). Herceptin also falls into the second grouping comprised of agents that target HER2, which is overexpressed in breast carcinoma and is associated with higher mortality in these patients. Hormone-type drugs that target receptor positive cancers, such as tamoxifen for estrogen receptor positive breast cancer and anti-androgens in receptor-positive prostate cancer, also affect growth-stimulatory pathways.

DESIGN OF CLINICAL TRIALS WITH MOLECULARLY TARGETED THERAPIES

The selection of the appropriate patient population is of utmost importance for **trials with molecularly targeted therapies**. Knowledge of the exact target of the therapy and assays to assess whether each individual possesses this target are also crucial for evaluation. Selection of the proper dosage to administer is important, but sometimes difficult in trials of molecularly targeted therapies. The dose is usually chosen on the basis of whether it attains desired plasma levels and regulates the target. The effects of the agent on the target must be measured. For tumors, this requirement often presents a problem in terms of procurement of appropriate samples for examination. Thus, surrogate markers are often measured, or imaging studies are performed as substitutes. Success needs to be defined for a trial because agents directed against one particular target may produce changes but not lead to complete abrogation of the tumor cells. This is why most cancer treatments are a combination of modalities.

HORMONE THERAPY

Hormone therapy in cancer treatment works by slowing or stopping the growth of hormone-sensitive tumors. This is accomplished either by **interference** with the action of the hormone or by **blocking** the body's ability to produce hormones. Tumors that are not hormone sensitive will not be affected by hormone therapy. In the treatment of hormone-sensitive breast cancer, ovarian suppression agents such as goserelin acetate or leuprorelin may be utilized. Ovarian suppression agents work by interfering with the signals the pituitary gland sends to the ovaries to produce estrogen. In the treatment of prostate cancer, antiandrogens may be used in combination with an orchiectomy or in combination with a luteinizing hormone–releasing hormone agonist. Antiandrogens work by competing with androgens for binding to the androgen receptor, thereby decreasing the ability of the androgens to promote or accelerate prostate cancer growth. Examples of antiandrogen agents include flutamide, enzalutamide, bicalutamide, and nilutamide.

HORMONES, ANTI-HORMONES, AND THEIR INHIBITORS FOR CANCER TREATMENT

A number of **anti-hormonal agents** are used for the treatment of specific cancers. These agents act by competing for hormonal receptor sites. Steroids are fatty compounds containing four carbon ring structures, and many hormones (particularly the sex hormones, such as androgens and estrogens) are steroids. Steroidal and non-steroidal structured anti-hormones are employed in treatment of cancers like prostate cancer (for example flutamide or Eulexin) and breast cancer (most commonly tamoxifen or Nolvadex). There are a number of aromatase inhibitors available as well, which block the conversion of androgens to estrogens. Prednisone is a commonly administered corticosteroid used to reduce inflammation and control certain immune responses. While it is used primarily for pain management, it is often given to patients with lymphoid malignancies. Reagents related to the hormonal system also include luteinizing hormone antagonists for chemical castration in prostate cancer, steroidal progestational drugs, and somatostatin inhibitors.

Localized Therapy

LOCALIZED THERAPY

Localized cancer therapy is targeted directly at the location of the malignancy in attempt to minimize damage to the surrounding tissue. There are three main **types of localized cancer therapy**:

- **Intravesical**: Chemotherapy is instilled in liquid form directly into the bladder via catheter. The medication remains in the bladder for up to 2 hours and then is drained. This route is most commonly used for bladder cancer after a transurethral resection of a bladder tumor and targets only the cells lining the bladder. Mitomycin is the most common drug used in intravesical chemotherapy. Gemcitabine and Valrubicin can also be used.
- **Intraperitoneal**: Chemotherapy is instilled directly into the peritoneal space through an access port that is placed prior to treatment near the rib cage. The fluid remains in the peritoneal cavity for about 1-2 hours, with the patient changing positions every fifteen minutes, and is then drained. The drug can also be administered directly after a tumor debulking surgery via Hyperthermic Intraperitoneal Chemotherapy (HIPEC). In this case the drug is instilled during surgery, then the surgical site is closed and the chemotherapy is absorbed into the cavity. This route is commonly used for cancers within the GI tract in addition to ovarian cancer.
- **Intrathecal**: Chemotherapy is administered into the cerebrospinal fluid (CSF) that flows around the brain and spinal cord. This can also be used prophylactically. The drugs are administered via lumbar puncture or through a shunt called an Ommaya reservoir. This is the only possible route of chemotherapy for cancers that have entered the CSF.

Surgical Treatment and Symptom Management

SURGERIES USED FOR VARIOUS PURPOSES

Surgery can be used for various purposes for the cancer patient:

- **Prophylactic purposes**: The excision of premalignant lesions
- **Diagnostic purposes**: Biopsies for definitive histological diagnosis
- **Staging purposes**: The extent of the carcinoma must actually be observed inside the patient
- **Treatment purposes**: The simple removal of the entire carcinomatous tumor for curative reasons
- **Palliation purposes**: Not for altering the outcome of the disease, but to maintain the best quality of life for the patient and to allow death with dignity and maximum comfort

SURGERY USED FOR CANCER TREATMENT

When cancer is first suspected, **surgery** is used to establish a diagnosis. This is accomplished through many types of biopsies. **Incisional biopsy** can be performed where a small sample of suspected tissue is removed for testing, or **excisional biopsy** can be performed in which the entire suspected tissue is removed. Biopsy can also be accomplished using a needle with a fine point or larger size to perform a core biopsy. Lymph nodes can also be biopsied using a needle technique. Surgery is used to determine how advanced the disease has become and to stage the disease. This involves removing the malignant tissue and obtaining tissue samples from multiple areas to assess for the presence of disease. Surgery can also be used as a primary **treatment** of the disease with removal of the affected organs. This is accomplished by removing the malignant tumor. Surgery can also help to **debulk** a tumor and reduce symptoms, though this does not cure the disease and is performed as a palliative treatment.

TYPES OF CANCER SURGERY

Types of cancer surgery include the following:

- **Surgical excision** is done to remove the malignant tissue. This involves the removal of just the involved tissue with a margin of healthy tissue, or it may be more extensive and include removal of the affected tissue and surrounding lymph nodes and other tissues.
- **Electrosurgery** involves applying an electric stimulus to the area affected by the malignancy and destroying the cancer cells.
- **Cryosurgery** can be performed, which involves applying liquid nitrogen to the cancer tissues. This causes destruction of the malignant cells through a freezing process.
- **Laser treatments** can be applied directly to the malignant tissue to cause destruction of the malignant cells. This is performed using a specialized scalpel that emits laser stimulus.
- **Stereotactic surgery** is used with brain tumors to provide an exact location of the tumor in a three-dimensional appearance. Special equipment is used for positioning the patient to utilize this type of surgery.

Surgery can be performed through a scope approach with laparoscopy and endoscopy. Both biopsy and removal of tumors can be performed utilizing this approach.

SURGICAL ANATOMIC CHANGES RESULTING IN IMPAIRMENTS IN VENTILATION

Surgery may be done to remove a section of a lung, or the entire lung, which is invaded by cancer. This decreases the amount of **oxygen** that can be inspired with each breath. During the post-op period the patient may have a chest tube present, which will also affect **lung expansion** during breathing. Cancer involving the chest wall may require removal of ribs and muscle tissue, which will impair a patient's ability to take deep breaths.

Patients who have cancer of the trachea may require surgical excision of the tumor. This may result in a permanent **tracheostomy site** which requires special care and serves as another path through which air can escape before reaching the lungs.

Frequent surgeries that are performed on patients with lung cancer include a **pneumonectomy** to completely remove a lung, a **lobectomy** to remove one lobe of a lung, or various-sized **resections** to take just a small portion of the lung.

SURGICAL SYMPTOM MANAGEMENT
COLOSTOMIES

A colostomy involves the creation of a hole through the abdomen to connect with a portion of the colon. This is usually created after a portion of the colon is removed because of invasive cancer. A colostomy can be temporary or permanent.

- **Temporary colostomies** are created when it is believed that the colon will be able to function normally in the future and the patient will once again be able to have regular bowel movements. This is used after a tumor is removed that is causing obstruction of the colon or to allow a temporary diversion for stool while the bowel mends after surgery is performed.
- A **permanent colostomy** is created when a large enough portion of the bowel is removed that it is believed the patient will no longer be able to have regular bowel movements on their own. This usually occurs when a tumor invades the area from the colon and distally.

STOMAS

- **End stomas** are created by cutting the bowel and then diverting it through the abdominal wall. The rest of the bowel that is left distally may be removed from the body or sewn off.
- **Loop stomas** involve bringing a section of the colon out through an incision in the abdomen. This is usually a temporary situation when a bowel obstruction is present or to help with symptom treatment at the end of a patient's battle with cancer. Another surgical procedure can be performed in the future to correct the colostomy so that the bowel will function normally.
- **Double-barrel stomas** are two stomas present in the abdominal wall. The stoma that is formed from the proximal portion of bowel will excrete stool while the distal portion only secretes mucus. The consistency of the stool from the proximal end will vary depending on its location. If more distal in the bowel, the proximal stoma will secrete stool that is more formed, but if more proximal in the bowel, the stool will be more watery.

URINARY DIVERSIONS

A urinary diversion is a surgical re-routing of the flow of urine so that urine is usually no longer excreted through the urethra, but rather through another opening or through the abdominal wall, usually into a collecting device.

Urinary diversions are needed when urine flow is **blocked**. Common reasons for blockage include: birth defects to the urinary system, kidney or bladder stones, trauma to the urethra, an enlarged prostate, or tumors in the pelvic cavity. A diversion may be needed when cancer invades the bladder and a cystectomy, or bladder removal, is necessary.

When a patient has a urinary diversion, they should be assessed for any changes in skin integrity because of the potential for skin breakdown when urine is in contact with it.

URINARY DIVERSION TYPES

There are two major types of diversions:

- **Incontinent urinary diversions** are diversions that do not allow the patient to have control over the times at which they void. They are connected to a drainage bag, and urine generally drains into the bag as it is made. Incontinent diversions are created from a portion of the small intestine. A stoma is created with the small intestine, and the ureters are attached to the section of intestine to drain urine from the body. Urinary reflux can occur and the patient is at a high risk for developing infections in the urinary tract. This also places the patient at an increased risk of developing kidney infections.
- **Continent urinary diversions** are diversions which allow the patient to have control of when they will void. One way to create this type of diversion involves connecting the ureters from the kidneys to a section of the large intestine. This allows urine to flow through the intestine and colon to be exited through the anus. A valve is created which allows the patient to maintain continence.
  - **Orthotopic neobladders** are a type of continent diversion. These involve making a bladder from a portion of the stomach or intestine and connecting the ureters to it to collect urine. The urethra is also attached to enable urine to flow normally out of the body. This procedure is usually performed when there is bowel disease or damage from disease.

SURGICAL MANAGEMENT OF LYMPHEDEMA

Surgical intervention is indicated for the alleviation of lymphedema when:

- Medical procedures have failed.
- The swelling is extreme enough to prevent use of the limb.
- There are significant skin changes.
- Infection of the area persists.

The primary goals of specific procedures are either to reinstate proper fluid drainage or to reduce the size of the limb by removing tissue and fat. One physiologic approach to the reestablishment of proper drainage is to build a lymphatic bridge through use of flaps made from skin, omentum, or small bowel tissue. There are a number of microsurgical procedures available. Two of these involve anastomoses, or the surgical unions of two parts: (1) lymphaticovenous anastomosis (LVA), which bypasses the obstruction by joining the lymphatic to a vein, and (2) lymphatic-lymphatic anastomosis (L-L), which avoids local areas of obstruction by creating new lymphatic connections. Both have been relatively successful in reducing lymphedema. A third procedure called a lymph nodal-venous shunt is also occasionally done.

Most **excisional procedures** for surgical management of lymphedema strive to remove skin layers and subcutaneous tissue where most lymphedema is localized. Some of these, like the Charles procedure, also resurface the skin with a graft. Since there is fat deposition in lymphedema, liposuction is sometimes done to debulk the area of fat and fluids, usually in conjunction with more conservative methods, such as compression. Although it is not standard practice in the United States, adjunctive use of daily hyperthermia of the affected limb has been used effectively in China. Medical management, surgery, and other procedures are often combined for overall optimal management.

Radiation Therapy

TARGET THEORY OF RADIATION

Target theory states that radiation damage results from direct and indirect hits on the DNA chain. Ionization affects either the molecules of the cell or the cell environment. As a result of direct hits:

1. There is a change or loss of a **base** (thymine, adenine, guanine, or cytosine).
2. Then there is a breakdown of the **hydrogen bond** between the two chains of the DNA molecule.
3. There are breaks in one or both chains of the **DNA molecule.**
4. **Cross-linking** of the chains occurs after breakage.

These four events lead to mutations that lead to impaired cellular function or cell death of the cancer cells. An indirect hit refers to the ionization of water, the medium surrounding the molecular structures within the cell, which causes a change in the cellular environment.

ELECTROMAGNETIC RADIATION

Electromagnetic radiation is energy traveling through space while generating electric and magnetic force fields. There are basically two types of electromagnetic radiation: **gamma rays** that are discharged from disintegrating radioactive nuclei, and **x-rays** that are emitted from outside the nucleus without mass or electrical charge. Electromagnetic radiation can be described as either discrete bundles or particles of energy called photons, or in terms of wave propagation. Each type of radiation travels at the speed of light, but the wavelength, or distance between the same phases in adjoining waves differs and is distinctively characteristic for different types of electromagnetic radiation. Waves with shorter wavelengths (such as x-rays) also have higher frequencies or a higher number of wave cycles per second, and their energy is disseminated in discrete massless parcels called photons.

RADIATION PHYSICS AND RADIOBIOLOGY

Radiation physics is the study of the effects of radiation exposure on cells. Radiation treatment for cancer involves treating malignancies with a focused beam of ionizing radiation. This causes changes within the cancer cells that result in their destruction. Ionizing radiation can be electromagnetic or particulate. **Electromagnetic radiation** is effective using energy waves. An example of this is a regular x-ray. **Particulate radiation** involves the smallest elements of cells, such as electrons, protons, and neutrons.

Radiobiology is the study of the living cell after radiation treatment has been applied to the cell. It examines the specific actions that occur to promote cell destruction, as well as the length of time necessary for this to occur. It also examines the various doses necessary to destroy cells, with the minimum dosage required to destroy a cell effectively being the most desirable. It also examines the effects that radiation treatment has on normal tissues.

ROLES OF RADIATION IN CANCER TREATMENT AND MANAGEMENT

Radiation can play several roles in cancer treatment and management:

- **Cure**: Radiation treatment for a cure has a primary goal of eliminating all cancer cells so that growth of the cancer cannot occur. It is also hoped that normal, non-cancerous cells will not be damaged from radiation exposure.
- **Control**: While a cure is not the expected outcome, the radiation treatment should control further development of cancer cells. This allows the patient to be without symptoms of the cancer.
- **Adjuvant**: This type of radiation treatment is performed before surgery to decrease the size of a tumor and make it more easily resected, or it is performed after surgery to destroy any remaining cancer cells that may be present.
- **Palliation**: This type of radiation treatment is aimed at helping to control the symptoms from cancer. This is done when there is no hope for a cure, but the patient is experiencing unpleasant symptoms from the disease, such as pain. The goal is to make the patient more comfortable.

UNITS OF RADIATION USED IN RADIATION ONCOLOGY

Wilhelm Conrad Roentgen has been credited as the discoverer of x-rays in 1895. He observed fluorescence on papers in the room where he was performing experiments passing electricity through high-vacuum tubes. He used this phenomenon to take the first radiograph of his wife's hand. Therefore, the roentgen unit was established in 1928 in his honor. The **roentgen**, or **R**, is a **unit of radiation exposure**; however, it does not necessarily reflect the actual radiation dose delivered to the tissues. Newer units represent the amount of ionizing radiation absorbed by the tissue. These units include the following:

- **Radiation absorbed dose (rad)** = 100 ergs absorbed per gram of tissue. Note: rad and rem (roentgen-equivalent man) are interchangeable terms, and in soft tissues they are roughly equivalent to roentgen units.
- **Gray (Gy) or sievert (Sv) units** = 100 rads = 1 joule absorbed per kg of tissue.

The quantification of dose absorbed is more important than exposure, because it corresponds to potential biological destruction.

RADIATION AND DELIVERY METHODS UTILIZED IN CLINICAL SETTINGS

Radiation used in clinical settings is delivered by one of three methods:

- First, there is **external beam radiation**, which uses an outside source and is directed at the desired tissues. This type of therapy typically employs either x-rays generated by linear accelerators or gamma rays that are emitted through nuclear radioactive decay.
- Second, there is a variation of external beam therapy, called **teletherapy**, which uses high intensity Cobalt-60 as a source of high-energy gamma rays.
- The third type of radiation therapy is **brachytherapy**, in which a source of radiation is introduced inside the patient. The radioactive isotopes used for brachytherapy emit particles from the nucleus as they decay. The particles are usually alpha (α) or beta (β), possessing either positive charges (α and β^+) or a negative charge (β^-). They are taken in at the site, in process of which gamma rays are also given off.

All of these types constitute low linear energy transfer or LET radiation, which means they only ionize a small proportion of the tissues they pass through.

111

CLINICALLY USEFUL ISOTOPES THAT PRODUCE RADIATION BY RADIOACTIVE DECAY

Photons or gamma rays of radiation are emitted from the nucleus of an isotope as it goes from an unstable to a more stable form (a process referred to as "radioactive decay"). The clinical utility of this nuclear disintegration depends upon: 1) the half-life of the isotope (the time needed for half the population to decay), 2) the mean energy of the gamma ray in kiloelectron volts (KEV), and 3) the absence of other undesired byproducts. The **five major isotopes**, in descending order of gamma ray energy emitted, and their major uses are as follows:

1. Cesium (Cs)-137: Women's reproductive organ implants.
2. Gold (Au)-198: Its very short half-life limits its use.
3. Iridium (Ir)-192: Used in numerous types of implants.
4. Iodine (I)-125: Widely used, especially for prostate implants.
5. Palladium (Pd)-103: Primarily utilized in prostate implants.

In addition, Radon (RA)-126 was once employed for implants, but its half-life is too long (1620 years), and it gives off radioactive radon gas. Cobalt (Co)-60 releases very high energy gamma rays, which makes it useful for external beam teletherapy. There are also a number of other clinically utilized isotopes that emit beta particles, in particular Strontium (Sr)-90.

CLINICALLY USEFUL RADIATION PRODUCED WITH A LINEAR ACCELERATOR

In a **linear accelerator**, high-frequency electromagnetic waves called microwaves are used to accelerate or speed up electrons that are aimed at a target, usually tungsten. Some of the rapidly moving electrons reach and interact with the electromagnetic field of the tungsten nucleus, producing high-energy x-rays called bremsstrahlung or braking energy x-rays. The accelerator usually has other parts beyond the target to direct the x-ray beam (collimators) and to produce a homogeneous beam (flattening filters). The x-ray beam is aimed at the tumor tissue to be treated. The x-rays produced in a linear accelerator have sufficient energy levels to spare tissue through which they pass or to travel through outer tissue types (such as skin) without much interaction, thus targeting the desired tissues. Normal x-ray machines, such as those used to make radiographs, produce much lower energy x-rays utilizing a different mechanism. Specifically, they eject an electron from an inner orbital shell, which is then replaced with one from an outer shell to produce an x-ray with energy characteristic of the compound used.

ALTERNATIVE MODALITIES FOR RADIOTHERAPY
INTENSITY-MODULATED RADIOTHERAPY

Intensity-modulated radiotherapy (IMRT) is a method of delivering radiation preferentially to tumor areas while obscuring other normal tissues, thus theoretically augmenting the therapeutic ratio. This obscuration is achieved by utilization of various radiation beam intensities delivered from different planes. The beams are usually regulated by using multi-leaf collimators to change intensities and alter the planes. Other alternatives include serial tomotherapy, which uses narrow slit beams during rotation of the patient, and combinations of photon and electron beams. In contrast to conventional treatment plans, the planning is done in inverse order. In other words, computers optimize various parameters based on the desired outcome or dose distribution. This is a newer technique and has not been well-studied.

PARTICLE RADIATION THERAPY

Particle radiation therapy uses high linear energy transfer particles for radiation treatment, instead of traditional x-rays or gamma rays. In theory, the higher energy of the particles should have a higher kill rate for hypoxic cells. It should also circumvent the cell cycle, and less damage repair should occur. There are two types of particle radiation therapy. In the first, neutron therapy, high energy neutron beams are delivered. This modality is not used very often because it has been proven effective for only a few malignancies, such as salivary gland tumors and some sarcomas, and it can produce late-onset toxicity. Positively charged protons are also used for particle radiation therapy. Their energy level is less than that of neutrons and slightly more than the energy of conventional x-rays. The main advantage of proton therapy is that the energy is slowly absorbed in outer tissue layers until it reaches its maximum, termed the Bragg peak. Maximum absorption is generally at deeper sites than reached by x-rays. The absorption of energy then quickly plummets, which makes this method ideal for malignancies that are in propinquity (i.e., in close proximity) to other vital structures.

FRACTIONATED RADIOTHERAPY

Fractionation is the division of total radiation administered into smaller fractions. Its use is based on several principles. In theory, splitting up radiation doses should allow normal tissues to be spared, or to repopulate during the interim when sub-lethal DNA damage is being repaired. The division should also give the tumor cells time to accumulate or reassert into radiosensitive phases of the cycle, especially if reoxygenation has occurred. Early-responding tumors like those involving the bone marrow or mucosal tissues, as well as normal tissues, are able to proliferate and repopulate more quickly than late responders. The early responders are also more susceptible to toxicity. The late responding population tends to be cells that are terminally differentiated and have no stem cell precursors available, such as connective tissues and the spinal cord. These tumor cells experience toxicity related only to overall dosage, and their response is late.

INTERACTION OF X-RAYS WITH MATTER

Depending on the energy level of the x-ray and the makeup of the matter (i.e., the target tissue for cancer treatment), there are up to five possible ways the two can interact. Two of these contribute significantly in the design of radiation therapy strategies:

- First, if an x-ray photon is able to reach the firmly bound inner shell orbit electrons of the target tissue, a type of interaction called the "**photoelectric effect**" can occur. Here, the photon's energy is absorbed by the inner shell electron, which is subsequently ejected as an x-ray with a characteristic energy level. This photoelectric effect is exploited in diagnostic radiology, but it is problematic in therapeutic settings because it is non-selective.
- Second, if the original photon is not completely absorbed and is instead dispersed at various angles, a series of interactions and ionizations can occur. This phenomenon is called **Compton scattering**, and it is the most useful for therapy because most of the ejected electrons are in the outer orbital shells. Thus, they bounce off and produce ionizations numerous times, and many tissue types are affected.

Besides the photoelectric effect and Compton scattering, three other types of interactions between x-rays and matter might occur. One is called "**coherent scattering**." While not commonly observed in therapeutic settings, it may be described as the change of direction (but without alteration of energy levels) that occurs when lower energy electrons strike against matter. Two other kinds of interactions can occur, both involving very high energy photons that enter the nucleus:

- One is called **pair production**, which occurs when the photon disappears and two subsequent species result—an electron and a positron. This does not usually present a problem in therapy, because the energies utilized are too low.
- The other is called **photodisintegration**. Here, the nucleus partially breaks up and neutrons are emitted. The clinical significance of this type of scattering is that it can be carcinogenic.

113

WAYS IN WHICH RADIATION CAN KILL CELLS IN TARGET TISSUES

Many of the effects of radiation on target cells are believed to involve damage to DNA, which eventually induces **cell death or apoptosis**. These types of effects can be either direct or indirect. In a direct effect, the DNA takes in the radiation, becomes ionized, and then is damaged in a way that prevents cell proliferation. In an indirect effect, adjacent water molecules are ionized to produce various types of highly reactive free radicals, which in turn interact with the DNA. The most significant type of damage to DNA is postulated to be double-strand breakage which eventually leads to cell death during mitosis. Radiation can also halt the cell cycle at various points, particularly during G1 and G2, or shift them into terminal differentiation; the result is that the cells cannot cycle or propagate. Radiation can induce changes that interrupt mitosis as well.

EFFECTS OF RADIATION THERAPY ON CELL CYCLE PHASE

Cells in either **late G2 or mitosis phases** are those most likely to be killed during exposure to radiation, while cells in the stages just prior to this (**early G2 and middle or late S phase**) are those least affected. The differences are probably related to the relative efficiency of DNA repair during different parts of the cell cycle. Two **transitions in the cell cycle** are also affected by radiation treatment, specifically, the conversion from the G2 to M phase and the switch from the G1 to S phase. The block at the G2 transition appears to be dose dependent.

EFFECTS OF OXYGENATION ON RESPONSE OF CELLS TO RADIATION

Cells that are highly oxygenated are about three times as likely to be killed with radiation compared to those that are not. Water molecules liberate free radicals that induce chemical reactions damaging DNA; these DNA changes cannot be efficiently repaired in the presence of oxygen because it is used to form permanent peroxides that cannot be reduced. Unfortunately, the percentage of cells falling into the hypoxic category is higher for tumor cells than for normal cell types. Theoretically this limits the effectiveness of radiation. Tumor cell hypoxia is common because tumors are inclined to outgrow their blood supplies, leaving oxygen in short supply. Even so, some animal studies have shown that reoxygenation can occur during radiation therapy. This occurs as some cells die and the tumor shrinks, bringing the remaining cells closer to the blood supply. If humans respond similarly, then theoretically long, multiple bouts of radiation are indicated to provide time between fractions for reoxygenation. Other ways to increase oxygen availability at tumor sites are being studied as well.

APPROACHES TO AFFECT OXYGENATION LEVELS

Various ways of radiosensitizing or increasing oxygen levels in tumor cells have been tried. In general, animal studies have been easier to control than human clinical trials, but these approaches may prove useful. Chemicals that attract the electrons produced during ionization, like nitroimidazole, have proven effective in animal models. Halogenated pyrimidines, which substitute halogens like bromine or iodine for the methyl group, have also been tried in an attempt to induce double-strand DNA breaks during irradiation. The most common approach is to use certain chemotherapeutic agents in combination with radiation therapy.

There are several compounds that can act as radioprotectors to reduce toxicity to normal cells. Radioprotectors typically have free sulfhydryl (SH) groups that are used to either absorb free radicals or aid in DNA repair by contribution of the hydrogen. Both radiosensitizers and radioprotectors can be incorporated into radiation protocols.

DETERMINATION OF X-RAY DOSAGES TO DELIVER DURING RADIATION THERAPY

X-rays produced by a linear accelerator have to travel through other tissues before reaching their target tissue. Most clinically useful photon energy ranges from 6-18 megaelectron volts (MeV), and is able to spare the skin and other relatively superficial tissue types. As the beam penetrates deeper into the tissues, it interacts with increasing numbers of electrons until it reaches a point where the maximum number of ionization events can occur and radiation effects are maximal. This point is referred to as **D_{max}**. Beyond the D_{max} plane, the photon beam becomes attenuated or weaker. Thus, given a known depth for the target tissue, the most important consideration is the energy level of the emitted x-ray beam. This is because the D_{max} plane is theoretically deeper as the MeV is increased. Other factors must also be taken into consideration, including the size of the beam, efficiency of scatter control, and the density of the tissue involved.

RELATIONSHIP BETWEEN ABSORBED DOSE OF RADIATION AND SURVIVING FRACTION OF CELLS

After exposure to radiation, irradiated cells are observed in various stages. The surviving fraction of cells at a given time can be monitored and a survival curve generated. In general, the **relationship between dose absorbed and surviving fraction is semi-logarithmic**. This means the fraction surviving is in reverse logarithmic proportion to the linear amount of the dose received. Dosage in Gy is plotted on the x-axis versus the logarithm of the surviving fraction on the y-axis. As the dosage increases, the curves become less uniform, with bending sections appearing. The exact reason for this bending is undetermined. For most clinically utilized radiation doses, the dose response curve can be described as having a linear-quadratic relationship.

TOLERATED RADIATION DOSE RANGES FOR COMMONLY TREATED MALIGNANCIES

Tolerated radiation dose ranges for commonly treated malignancies are those that typically do not reach the threshold for toxicity to the organ. The lowest tolerance dose is only 200 cGy for testicular cancer, before possible sterility. Other tolerance doses are much higher, up to 5000 to 6500 cGy, for brain, spinal cord, skin, stomach, rectal, esophageal, bladder and ovarian cancers, as well as certain eye damage. Still other types of malignancies can be treated with slightly lower doses before toxicity is likely to become an issue. Many of these toxic effects will affect functionality in significant ways, such as sterility for reproductive cancers, paralysis for spinal cord malignancies, and hemorrhaging for stomach or rectal cancer overdoses.

TYPICAL AND NON-STANDARD RADIATION FRACTIONATION SCHEMES

In the United States, a **typical or standard radiation fractionation scheme** is the administration of 1.8-2.0 Gy per day, five days a week for seven weeks. A common variation is to divide the size of the fraction, and thus individual treatment time, into twice-a-day administrations at half the dose. When late-responding tumors, like those in the spinal cord, are being treated, an altered scheme is used in which fewer but larger fractions (for example, five large 20 Gy fractions) are given. This makes sense because these types of tumors respond only to total dosage administered, not treatment length.

Two additional types of **altered schemes** are generally employed to avoid late tissue damage. Hyperfractionation schemes use smaller doses several times a day. While the overall treatment time is relatively unchanged, the total radiation given is slightly increased. Accelerated fractionation cuts down the total treatment time in order to thwart repopulation. These types of schemes change the number of daily fractions given, the fraction size, or total the dosage given. A variant is the accelerated boost protocol, in which a standard scheme is followed for the first four weeks, and multiple fractions are given for two additional weeks.

CELLULAR REPAIR MECHANISMS

A portion of irradiated cells will recover after each dose is given, generally within a 6-hour time frame. While the exact mechanism is unclear, DNA damage is apparently being repaired in these cells, allowing them to continue growing. There are **two types of repair** possible:

- The first type is the **repair of sub-lethal or less than complete damage**. This is evidenced by the observation of a broad shoulder on the survival curve of some cells and the fact that two widely spaced radiation doses may not be as effective as one larger one. Tissues that tend to respond later to radiation also may have a subpopulation of cells that can repopulate before further treatment.
- Another type of repair is **potentially-lethal damage repair**, in which the potential for killing the cell depends on its state—including cell cycle phase at the time of irradiation.

SET UP OF RADIATION FIELDS FOR TREATMENTS

Computed tomography (CT) is usually used for **radiation treatment evaluation and planning**, although sometimes MRI or PET scans are substituted. The best method is the direct transfer of CT images to a special software-enabled computer. There the clinician can delineate the tumor volume and other important structures using a range of CT slices, creating a three-dimensional view. After this, different tumor volumes are drawn: the gross tumor volume (GTC), as previously observed; the clinical tumor volume (CTV), which includes important adjacent structures such as lymphatic drains; and the planning tumor volume (PTV), which includes a further margin to account for variability of technique. Then all components of the radiation beam, such as number, energy level, angles, and shielding of normal tissues through use of collimators, are calculated and observed digitally on a simulated radiograph. At this juncture, the treatment plan can be instituted. However, for each treatment, the patient must be positioned exactly as he or she was for the initial development of the plan.

Bone Marrow/Stem Cell Transplants

BONE MARROW TRANSPLANTS

A bone marrow transplant is the infusion of bone marrow into a patient who has been treated previously with high dose chemotherapy or radiation to halt rejection of the transplanted material.

Types of **bone marrow transplants** include the following:

- **Allogenic**: Infusion of bone marrow from one individual to another.
- **Autologous**: Infusion of a patient's own bone marrow previously removed and stored.
- **Syngeneic**: Infusion from one identical twin to another.

ALLOGRAFTING VS AUTOGRAFTING FOR BONE MARROW TRANSPLANTS

Allografting is the process by which bone marrow is obtained from a donor and transplanted into the cancer patient. This can also be done with blood stem cells or umbilical cord blood that has been stored. Specialized tests need to be completed to confirm that the donor and patient will be a match to prevent a rejection reaction by the recipient. Identical twins are ideal donors for each other, but other family members or donor bone marrow may be used if the match is close enough.

Autografting of bone marrow involves removing bone marrow cells from the patient and returning the cells to them. This can be performed if a matched donor cannot be found. It is also used in patients who are at increased risk for developing a rejection reaction to donor bone marrow. There is a risk of the bone marrow cells containing cancer cells, so this needs to be ruled out before this procedure can be performed.

POTENTIAL COMPLICATIONS FROM BONE MARROW TRANSPLANTATIONS

Potential complications from bone marrow transplantations include the following:

- **Graft-versus-host disease** occurs when the patient develops a rejection reaction to bone marrow received from a donor that may not be a perfect genetic match. This occurs in as many as one-half of bone marrow recipients. High doses of steroids as well as other medications that decrease immune reactions can be used to try and prevent this from happening.
- **Interstitial pneumonitis** is an inflammation in lung tissue. It is more common in those patients who received radiation treatments to the chest, treatment with bleomycin, or are carriers of the cytomegalovirus. These infections can be caused by viruses, bacteria, or fungi. Antimicrobial medications are used to treat this infection.

HEPATIC SINUSOIDAL OBSTRUCTION SYNDROME

Hepatic sinusoidal obstruction syndrome (SOS), previously known as **veno-occlusive disease**, is a life-threatening complication that occurs in 15-20% of hematopoietic stem cell transplant patients. It occurs when fibrous material accumulates, resulting in obstruction of venules in the liver, which in turn causes portal hypertension and destruction of the liver cells. Clinical manifestations include hyperbilirubinemia, weight gain, ascites, right upper quadrant pain, hepatomegaly, splenomegaly, and jaundice. SOS should be considered in any patient that has these symptoms after stem cell transplant, especially in the first three weeks. Veno-occlusive disease is treated by maintaining intravascular volume and renal perfusion and minimizing fluid accumulation. Prevention includes minimizing risk factors, such as decreasing exposure to hepatotoxic medications, and iron chelation for those patients who already have liver disease related to increased iron levels. Prevention also includes prophylaxis, usually with ursodeoxycholic acid for allogenic transplants, beginning the day before stem cell transplant and continuing three months after the procedure.

Photodynamic Therapy

BASICS OF PHOTODYNAMIC THERAPY

Photodynamic therapy (PDT) is a cancer treatment modality that uses a combination of systemic photosensitizer drugs and activation by non-ionizing radiation in the presence of oxygen. The interaction is classified as a photo-oxidative reaction. Most of the drugs are injected intravenously several hours or days before the photo-activation step, and studies indicate that these photosensitizer drugs are preferentially absorbed by tumor cells. When light is applied, the photosensitizer is excited and reactive oxygen species are generated, eventually leading to cell death. PDT is most useful for the treatment of superficial cancers, such as skin cancers and digestive or respiratory tract cancers, because non-ionizing radiation in the visible or near-infrared range cannot penetrate as deeply as wavelengths used for radiation therapy. Since PDT only reaches mucosal surfaces and serous membranes, deeper tissues remain unaffected.

PHOTOSENSITIZERS

The following are currently used **photosensitizers**:

- **Porfimer sodium (Photofrin)**: A hematoporphyrin derivative with excitation at 630 nm and a photosensitivity period of 4-6 weeks after administration. It has been approved and sanctioned by the FDA for intravenous administration in PDT for three types of indications.
    - First, it can be used for palliation of dysphasia, which is the difficulty swallowing that often accompanies obstructing esophageal cancer. Photofrin is approved for use with patients who fail to respond to previous Nd:YAG-type laser therapy.
    - Second, this drug is also approved for use in patients with late stage endobronchial lung cancer, for relief of airway obstruction and palliation of associated symptoms.
    - Third, it is also authorized for PDT use in patients with early microinvasive endobronchial lung carcinoma, as an alternative to radiation therapy or surgery. In these patients, the light is distributed through a cylindrical diffuser incorporated into a bronchoscope.
- **5-aminolevulinic acid (Levulan)**: A heme precursor, excited by blue light, with a photosensitivity period of about 1 day; it is the only drug applied topically instead of intravenously that is FDA-approved to treat actinic keratosis.
- **Meta-tetra(hydroxyphenyl)chlorin or mTHPC (Foscan)**: A chlorin, excited at 652 nm, active for 15 days (extremely active), approved in Europe for use with head and neck squamous cell carcinomas.
- **Motexafin lutetium (Lutrin)**: Aromatic metalloporphyrin, excitation at 732 nm, with a short photosensitive period (appears to be between 3 and 24 hours).
- **Other chlorin molecules**: SnET2 (660-664 nm, 2-3 week sensitive period), N-aspartyl chlorin or LS11 (664 nm, sensitivity period currently undetermined), 2-[1-hexyloxy-ethyl]-2-devinyl pyropheophorbide-a or HPPH (665 nm, 1-2 days).
- **Silicon phthalocyanine (Pc4)**: Excitation at 672 nm, duration about 1 day.

Newer, second-generation, photosensitizing drugs include **Metvix** (for non-hyperkeratotic actinic keratosis and basal cell carcinoma), **Foscan** (for advanced head and neck cancer), **Laserphyrin** (for early centrally located lung cancer), **Visudyne** (for age-related macular degeneration), and **Redaporfin** (for biliary tract cancer).

LIGHT SOURCE

In photodynamic therapy, the **light source** is a laser. If more than one type of photosensitizer is used in a particular clinical setting, then the appropriate diode for the drug must be used. This necessitates the use of either interchangeable diodes or one diode that can be tuned to different wavelengths. Generally, the light is delivered through attached optical fibers or applicators. The distance between the light source and the tissue being treated is related to the activation wavelength: higher wavelengths, such as those approaching the infrared region, will penetrate more deeply.

Fluence, the dose of light, is measured in units of joules of energy deposited per square centimeter (J/cm^2). A laser will have a particular **fluence rate**, which is expressed as either watts (W) or milliwatts (mW) per square centimeter. Even though some light will scatter, the dosage is usually calculated based on an amount delivered as follows:

$$\text{delivered fluence } \left(\frac{J}{cm^2}\right) = \text{fluence rate } \left(\frac{W}{cm^2}\right) \times \text{treatment time (s)}$$

EFFECTS OF PDT

PDT can cause direct **cellular damage** by the generation of reactive oxygen species, which oxidize various proteins and lipids in the cell, such as those found in the mitochondria and plasma or nuclear membranes. Each photosensitizer is excited for a very brief period of time, measured in microseconds, so the efficiency of direct cell killing with PDT is highly dependent upon the drug used and the fluence rate. If the photosensitizer is present in normal cells in close proximity, then they can be affected by PDT as well. These types of effects include damage to **vascular endothelial cells**, which can indirectly lead to tumor cell death by abrogation of the blood supply to the tumor. After photodynamic therapy, many types of **immune cells** rapidly flood into the area treated and an inflammatory reaction occurs. This immune cell influx eventually sets up immunity to the tumor, and studies suggest immunocompetent cells can even transfer this immunity. There may also be an induction of certain types of immunosuppression, such as inhibition of contact hypersensitivity.

APOPTOSIS OR NECROSIS

PDT can cause either **apoptosis** (programmed cell death) or **necrosis** (disruption of the cell and release of its contents). The outcome has been associated with various factors, such as the portion of the cell where the drug is localized, dosage, and type of tissue. Generally, higher doses increase the possibility of necrosis over apoptosis. Photosensitizers that accumulate in the mitochondria tend to induce apoptosis because the transmembrane potential has been lost, thus calcium accumulates in the cell and cytochrome c is released into the cytoplasm. Localization in other areas has also been associated with preferential apoptosis. Animal models and clinical trials suggest that PDT can affect expression of various proteins involved in the process of cell death.

CURRENT CLINICAL TRIALS FOR PREMALIGNANT CONDITIONS AND EARLY-STAGE CANCERS

Photodynamic therapy primarily affects superficial tissue layers and thus is an ideal candidate for the treatment of **premalignant conditions** and early-stage cancers. Consequently, current clinical trials are largely centered on abnormalities in the aerodigestive tract. Multiple courses of PDT are being tried for treatment of Barrett's esophagus, a condition where early changes in the esophagus cause difficulty swallowing, as well as early-stage esophageal cancer. Porfimer sodium is sanctioned by the FDA for treatment of Barrett's esophagus with high-grade dysplasia if surgery is a poor option. Some trials have also tested PDT in the management of carcinoma in situ and early-stage cancers in the head and neck areas. While there is some indication that photodynamic therapy is effective for these conditions, it is not FDA approved for any of them at present.

CURRENT CLINICAL TRIALS FOR MORE INVASIVE AND ADVANCED CANCERS

The use of PDT is being studied in a variety of **more invasive and advanced cancers**. In particular, a malignancy involving the pleural membrane, which lines the chest wall and covers the lungs, are of great interest. These include investigations with PDT in non-small cell lung cancer with pleural involvement and mesothelioma, a malignancy of the pleural surface which is associated with asbestos exposure and for which there is currently no cure. PDT has been used in conjunction with other treatment modalities for these cancers, but at present the utility of PDT remains equivocal. Tumors that metastasize to, or originate in, the peritoneal or abdominal lining are being studied as PDT candidates as studies show some promise in these areas. Trials utilizing PDT are also ongoing for advanced and recurrent head and neck cancers, skin cancers, a central nervous system tumor called malignant glioma, and prostate carcinoma.

Disease-Specific Treatment

LUNG CANCER
TREATMENT OF SMALL AND NON-SMALL CELL LUNG CANCERS

Since small cell lung cancer (SCLC) is an aggressive disease, surgical procedures are not useful and not generally performed. If the cancer is relatively limited, chemotherapy and irradiation of both the chest and brain (to prevent brain metastases) are done. Otherwise, several cycles of combination or multi-agent chemotherapy are tried but the prognosis is poor. For non-small cell lung cancer (NSCLC), **surgical resection** is usually effective for the early stages I and II. For stages IIIA and IIIB, indicating metastatic involvement, chemotherapy possibly combined with radiation is generally used either before surgery (IIIA) or as the treatment modality. If the latter patients also have a malignant pleural effusion, they are treated as stage IV. Stage IV patients are given combination chemotherapy, mainly to improve their quality of life. Individuals with recurrent NSCLC are also treated with combination chemotherapy.

Symptom control includes medications to control pain, nebulizer treatments to attempt to open the airways and assist with breathing, and steroids to control inflammation.

THORACOTOMY

A traditional thoracotomy for the treatment of lung cancer involves an open incision with skin closure via subcutaneous sutures of staples. A chest tube is inserted to facilitate fluid drainage and lung expansion. A minimally invasive procedure known as video-assisted thoracoscopy surgery (VATS) may also be an option for patients. Two to three smaller incisions are made into the chest wall and a videoscope and other small surgical tools are utilized. Patients undergoing traditional thoracotomy have a longer hospitalization, longer recovery time, and higher morbidity, and they experience more pain than those undergoing a VATS.

Postoperative care includes incisional care, pain management, and a bowel regimen to combat the constipation that goes along with opioid use, ambulation, and care of the chest tube. In addition, pulmonary hygiene should be performed aggressively to decrease the likelihood of pneumonia, atelectasis, and respiratory failure. Deep breathing in the postoperative period decreases the likelihood of pulmonary complications.

> **Review Video: Chest Tubes**
> Visit mometrix.com/academy and enter code: 696975

BREAST CANCER

SYSTEMIC TREATMENTS

The goal with systemic treatment is to treat the whole body in an attempt to destroy any cancer cells that may have migrated from the primary cancer site. **Chemotherapy** is the main type of systemic treatment that is used to treat breast cancer. Some of the more common chemotherapy drugs used to treat breast cancer include Cytoxan, Adriamycin, Taxol, and Mexate. Very often, multiple chemotherapy drugs will be given for more effective treatment. Most patients will receive 4-6 treatments with chemotherapy, if side effects are tolerable enough to continue treatment. Increasing the length or dose of treatment has not been found to be more effective in treating breast cancer. Men with breast cancer (early hormone receptor-positive breast cancer) should be given tamoxifen as an adjuvant according to the American Society of Clinical Oncology.

LOCALIZED TREATMENTS

Localized treatments for breast cancer involve surgery or radiation treatments. Localized treatment options for breast cancer include the following:

- **Surgical procedures** performed for breast cancer include lumpectomies, segmental resection, or mastectomies. Mastectomies can remove just the breast tissue (subcutaneous mastectomy), breast tissue plus some of the skin over the lesion (skin-sparing mastectomy), breast tissue plus skin and glands (total mastectomy), breast tissue and skin plus axillary lymph nodes (modified radical mastectomy), or breast tissue and skin along with lymph nodes and pectoral muscle (radical mastectomy). Sometimes just the first lymph node to be affected by the cancer (the sentinel node) is removed. This is still investigative, though.
- **Radiation treatments** may be done to ensure destruction of all cancer cells. It can be done along with chemotherapy or on its own. Radiation usually begins 2-4 weeks following surgery and may be done for palliative treatment of bony lesions. Side effects include irritation of the overlying skin, tissue and nerve damage, and fatigue.

MASTECTOMY POSTOPERATIVE CARE

Postoperative nursing care for a patient who has undergone a mastectomy for the treatment of breast cancer includes a combination of high priority interventions that focus on assessment, support, and patient education. Wound care and remobilization of the affected side are a focus of physical recovery. In the **immediate postoperative period**, the arm should be positioned so that it is slightly elevated. Exercises to regain full range of motion can begin within 3-5 days after surgery and should be gradually increased. The patient should be educated on the positioning and care of the arm on the affected side, drains, pain management, IV lines and tubing, and ambulation. Early ambulation and the importance of coughing and deep breathing should be emphasized. The incision should be assessed for inflammation, tenderness, swelling, and drainage. If the patient has a drain in place, the fluid should be assessed and measured and the drain secured to the skin or clothing. Patients may struggle with feelings of sadness at the loss of their breasts. Additionally, the patient may feel anxious while awaiting the final pathology of the breast tissue and learning about the possible involvement of more lymph nodes.

PROSTATE CANCER

MANAGEMENT OF LOCALIZED, EARLY, AND ADVANCED PROSTATE CANCER

Localized prostate cancer would be defined as falling into the TMN categories of T1 or T2. Usually, these individuals also have serum PSA levels of <10 ng/mL and a Gleason score in the range of 2-6. Patients falling into these categories are often just monitored carefully, but a radical retropubic prostatectomy may be performed.

If prostate cancer is **detected early**, the patient may have some options with treatment:

- **Surgery** can be performed for removal of the prostate and surrounding lymph nodes. In certain instances, the testicles can also be removed, which stops the production of testosterone and can help to decrease the progression of the disease. There are risks with surgery and the patient can develop incontinence or impotence following surgery.
- **Radiation** can be performed to destroy the cancer cells within the prostate gland. There is the risk of damage to surrounding healthy tissues, though. Radiation can also be delivered through brachytherapy in which radiation seeds are implanted within the prostate. Androgen deprivation has also been used as an adjunct to external beam radiation treatment. Radiation therapy can be utilized after prostatectomy if the disease recurs, usually monitored by assessing for rising PSA levels.
- **Cryosurgery** can be performed in which extreme cold is applied to the lesions on the prostate to destroy them.

With advanced prostate cancer, **hormonal treatments** may be given to reduce the amount of testosterone produced. The patient can develop feminizing side effects, such as enlargement of the breasts and hot flashes. However, if the disease progresses (usually indicated by rising PSA levels) systemic chemotherapy may be initiated.

POSTOPERATIVE NURSING CARE FOR A TURP

Postoperative nursing care for a patient who has undergone a **transurethral resection of the prostate** (TURP) includes a thorough and accurate assessment of the patient. Patients who have had a TURP are at risk of hemorrhage. Vital signs should be monitored closely and an accurate intake and output record maintained. The patient's **urinary catheter** should be assessed for patency regularly. Urinary catheters can become occluded with clots, which can increase the risk of hemorrhage. **Urine** should be assessed for color and character and recorded. Increasing fluids helps to decrease the burning sensation patients may feel with the urinary catheter and also lessens the chance for the development of a urinary tract infection. Patients may experience incisional pain, pain caused by bladders spasms, or abdominal cramping postoperatively. **Analgesics** and **nonsteroidal anti-inflammatory agents** are used to manage incisional pain. **Belladonna** and **opium suppositories** may be used for the management of bladder spasms.

COLORECTAL CANCER

Most patients undergo **surgical treatment** for colorectal cancer. The extent of the surgery depends on how much of the colon is affected by the malignancy.

- A **colostomy** may be required following surgery, and this may be permanent or temporary.
- **Radiation therapy** can also be used to treat colorectal cancer. This can be done before surgery to help shrink a tumor so that it can be surgically removed, or it may be done following surgery to destroy any cancer cells that may remain. Permanent tissue damage can result from radiation therapy, depending upon the dose and number of treatments.
- **Chemotherapy** is usually done along with radiation treatments. This is usually done if there is some extension of a malignancy beyond a localized tumor.
- Other medications are being studied to target growth factors and help the body develop antibodies against cancer-causing cells. These are still in the clinic phase.

POSTOPERATIVE NURSING CARE FOR A COLOSTOMY

Postoperative assessment of the cancer patient who has undergone a **colostomy** includes assessment of vital signs and lung and bowel sounds. The stoma site should be assessed for color and size. The stoma should appear pink and moist. Intake and output should be accurately recorded including drainage from a nasogastric tube, urinary catheter, and stoma. Coughing and deep breathing exercises should be encouraged as well as early ambulation. Pain should be proactively managed. A thorough skin assessment should be performed to ensure adequate wound healing. Body image and sexuality concerns are likely and should be discussed with the patient postoperatively. Sexual counseling should begin while the patient is in the hospital. Patients often struggle with viewing the stoma and learning to care for it. The nurse will need to provide the patient with education on ostomy care and supplies as well as dietary needs.

BRAIN TUMORS
TREATMENT OPTIONS

Treatment options for brain tumors include the following:

- **Surgical resection** is done to remove the tumor if possible. This is done through a procedure called a **craniotomy**. The same positioning techniques are used as with a biopsy, and all or as much of the tumor as possible is removed. Along with the malignant tumor, some healthy tissue may also be removed. The patient may suffer alterations in function in relation to the area of the brain in which the tumor is located and surgery is performed.
- **Radiation therapy** may be performed after surgery or may be used if surgery is not possible. Many brain tumors have microscopic strings of cancer cells that spread throughout the brain tissue but are not visible on MRI. Radiation is aimed at destroying any of these remaining cancer cells. This can cause edema of the surrounding brain tumor and destruction of some of the healthy brain tissue that remains.
- **Chemotherapy** can also be given, but it is not considered a primary therapy for malignant brain tumors.

POSTOPERATIVE NURSING CARE FOR A CRANIOTOMY

Postoperative care of the **craniotomy** patient is complex because the patient is at risk for a multitude of postoperative complications. A thorough and accurate **neurological assessment** is paramount. **Hemodynamic stability** is critical and should be regularly assessed. Hypertension in the postoperative craniotomy patient increases the risk of hemorrhage. Hypotension may cause hypoperfusion and brain ischemia. Postoperative interventions include DVT prophylaxis, incision and drain care, early ambulation, and prevention of atelectasis through incentive spirometry. Physical and occupational therapy should be involved in the evaluation and treatment of the patient postoperatively. Nursing staff should be aware of the risk of postoperative complications and assess the patient for early signs of these complications. Meningitis, brain abscess, and wound infection may manifest with signs and symptoms including fever, headache, malaise, redness, warmth or purulent drainage from the incision site, nausea and vomiting, and altered levels of consciousness. Additional complications may include endocrine complications such as diabetes insipidus or syndrome of inappropriate antidiuretic hormone secretion, postoperative hemorrhage, seizures, or a leak in cerebral spinal fluid.

PRIMARY OR SALVAGE THERAPY OF MELANOMAS

Primary **melanomas** are surgically excised. The margin around the site required is ascertained by the thickness of the melanoma and the area where it is located. A thicker lesion requires a larger excision margin, and some sites such as the fingers, toes, soles of the foot, or ears may necessitate other surgical procedures in conjunction. Sentinel nodes are often biopsied if regional lymph node involvement is not clinically evident. If regional nodes are metastatic, they are dissected. Patients who have large primary lesions or nodal involvement are generally also given interferon alpha or dacarbazine (DTIC), the only currently approved agents, or they may be enrolled in other clinical trials. These systemic adjuvants mainly alleviate symptoms. Once metastatic disease becomes systemic, patient survival is typically only about six to nine months.

NONMELANOMA SKIN CANCERS
BASIC FEATURES

About four out of every five cases of nonmelanoma skin cancer are **basal cell carcinoma (BCC)**, which usually presents as either a reddish ulcerated bump on the skin or as a lighter hardened plaque. Most other nonmelanoma skin cancers are **squamous cell carcinomas (SCC)**, which usually appear as raised areas that are either red or skin-toned and have ulcerations and patchy areas of hard horny tissue called keratoses.

Organ transplant patients are prone to develop SCC. Patients with SCC are more likely to develop metastases than those with BCC, although the latter can reoccur at the primary site. Lack of differentiation in either type can portend a more clinically aggressive tumor. There are other generally rare and often more aggressive malignancies that can emulate BCC or SCC that should be excluded via differential diagnosis such as sebaceous gland carcinoma and Merkel cell carcinoma.

MANAGEMENT

Primary basal cell or squamous cell carcinomas are generally surgically excised. A procedure called Mohs surgery is used in more aggressive or indistinct cases. Other approaches include radiation treatment, obliteration of the lesion by physical means, and administration of interferons or their activators. Once metastasis has occurred, treatment is generally multimodal, including surgery, radiation, and chemotherapy. Most people with nonmelanoma skin cancers have a much better chance of survival than those who present with melanoma. The prognosis for patients with either BCC or SCC is usually excellent, but if metastases develop in SCC cases, the individual has a less than 50% chance of surviving 5 years. The rarer skin cancers are associated with greater severity. Most skin cancers are associated with exposure to ultraviolet radiation, and there are available potential chemo preventive agents such as retinoids and COX-2 inhibitors.

ACUTE LYMPHOCYTIC LEUKEMIA (ALL)

Chemotherapy is also used to treat ALL. Cranial radiation is performed if the spread of the disease includes the central nervous system. Chemotherapy may be continued after remission is achieved and medications that were not used before may be used for this maintenance therapy.

Bone marrow transplant from a matched donor can also be performed to treat ALL. There is the risk of rejection of the donor marrow by the patient. Bone marrow transplants have been attempted in which the marrow is removed from the patient and the leukemic cells are removed before the marrow is replaced in the patient.

In children, the **maintenance therapy** of chemotherapeutic medications may continue for 2 to 3 years following remission. Bone marrow transplant can also be attempted in children. Using autologous bone marrow may not be an option for those patients with advanced disease.

Each of the chemotherapeutic agents has its own side effects and the patient should be educated on these potential effects.

ACUTE MYELOGENOUS LEUKEMIA (AML)

The primary treatment for AML is high dose **chemotherapy**. Survival rates are improving for patients with AML because of advances made in drug treatment of the disease. Some agents that are now produced not only work to destroy the leukemic cells, but also help to promote the growth and maturity of normal blood cells. If there is metastatic spread of the disease into the brain, radiation is often used to treat the cranial lesions.

Once remission is achieved, the chemotherapy agents that were originally used may be given once a month to provide maintenance therapy. This is to help prevent return of the disease and prolong the remission state.

Bone marrow transplant can be used if chemotherapy treatment does not prevent recurrence of the disease. About one-half of patients have a successful result from bone marrow transplant. A match must be found between a potential donor and a patient, and there is a risk of rejection by the patient.

CHRONIC MYELOGENOUS LEUKEMIA (CML)

Chemotherapy is the primary treatment used to treat CML. The most common drugs used are given orally and help to cure the disease by decreasing the production of white blood cells. If the disease worsens, chemotherapy doses are usually increased, but this does not usually result in better results.

CML can cause a condition called a **blastic crisis**. Repeat doses of chemotherapy may be used to treat this condition and radiation may also be used to help slow down the progression of any lesions forming within the bones. Chemotherapeutic medications may be given intrathecally to treat the development of disease within the central nervous system.

Bone marrow transplant can be used with approximately one-half of patients having successful long-term results. Autologous bone marrow transplant has varying results. Bone marrow transplant can be used to treat a blastic crisis, but this has not had extremely successful results.

CHRONIC LYMPHOCYTIC LEUKEMIA (CLL)

With CLL, the patient is not usually treated until they begin to exhibit symptoms from the disease. Some of the symptoms that warrant treatment included enlarged and painful lymph nodes, anemia, decreased blood counts, or enlarged liver or spleen.

- **Chemotherapy drugs** can be used to slow down the production of immature lymph cells and to decrease the production of leukemic lymph cells.
- **Steroids** may be helpful if the white blood cell count is elevated or if all cell types are decreased.
- In severe cases, the **spleen** may be removed if medications are not helpful in controlling symptoms.
- **Radiation** can be helpful when the spleen or lymph nodes are enlarged and causing pain. The aim of this treatment would be to decrease production of immature lymph cells.
- Right now, **bone marrow transplant** is not generally used to treat CLL but studies are being conducted to assess the effectiveness of this treatment.

CHILDHOOD LYMPHOMA

Variants of childhood non-Hodgkin lymphomas (NHL) are managed differently:

- **Burkitt's lymphoma** patients are generally managed with aggressive bouts of cyclophosphamide-based therapies. Treatment regimens for lymphoblastic lymphomas resemble those for ALL.
- **Large cell lymphomas** tend to be very heterogeneous, complicating treatment approaches, but various chemotherapeutic regimens are under investigation.
- Radiation and surgery are rarely utilized to treat **non-Hodgkin lymphomas**, whereas limited radiation may be employed in cases of **Hodgkin disease**. If the child has a larger tumor burden or a recurrence, his or her prognosis is poor.

Novel salvage approaches have included various drug combinations or high dose regimens as well as autologous hematopoietic stem cell transplantation.

HODGKIN LYMPHOMA

Treatment of Hodgkin lymphoma include the following:

- In the early stages of the disease, **radiation** alone can be tried to control the disease in localized areas. **Chemotherapy** may also be given in the early stages of disease followed by radiation treatment. Multiple chemotherapeutic agents may be given for the most effective treatment coverage.
- With more advanced disease, **chemotherapy** is the mainstay of treatment. This may be done alone or may be followed up with **radiation therapy**. Multiple chemotherapeutic medications may be given, especially with end-stage disease.
- For patients who have a relapse of multiple myeloma after a period of remission from Hodgkin lymphoma, different **chemotherapy** drugs from those used previously may be given. If the patient has been in remission for at least one year, the same medications that were used before may be given again. **Autologous bone marrow transplant** has proved effective in treating disease at this stage also. Though controversial, **blood stem cell treatments** are also very effective at inducing a remission state.

NON-HODGKIN LYMPHOMA

Treatment of non-Hodgkin lymphoma includes the following:
- Treatment is often delayed until the patient develops symptoms. In the early stages of non-Hodgkin lymphoma, **radiation treatments** are used in localized areas where the affected lymph nodes are present.
- **Chemotherapy** may also be used as a treatment. A medication that supplies antibodies against the disease may also be used to treat the disease.
- With advanced disease, multiple **chemotherapeutic medications** are used and **radiation** may be given at the same time. **Antibody medication** may also be given to try and induce a state of remission.
- In the patient who has a relapse of the disease after a state of remission, **chemotherapy** is frequently given using medications that have not been given in the past. **Stem cell treatments** are also effective at treating recurrent non-Hodgkin lymphoma.
- Treatment is usually quite aggressive with non-Hodgkin lymphoma and patients should be closely monitored for side effects from the multiple medications used to treat the disease.

MULTIPLE MYELOMA

Treatment for multiple myeloma includes the following:

- **Multiple myeloma** is treated with **chemotherapy**. **Steroids** are often frequently given with the chemotherapy medications. **Interferon** can also be used to decrease the production of plasma cells when bone marrow biopsy reveals elevated levels of plasma cells.
- If there is bony involvement with lesions present, **radiation treatment** may be performed and directed at the specific sites involved.
- **Stem cell treatment** has had excellent results with almost one-half of patients entering remission following treatments. This is most effective in patients under 70-years-old.
- **Bisphosphonates** such as Fosamax have shown some effectiveness at treating multiple myeloma when used in conjunction with standard treatments. This helps to promote calcium deposition in the bones to improve bone strength and decrease the risk of pathologic fractures.
- **Thalidomide** has been given to some patients who have not responded to other treatments of multiple myeloma. It works by decreasing the levels of certain proteins that are elevated with the disease.

CERVICAL CANCER

TREATMENT OPTIONS

There are a couple of factors to consider when deciding which treatment to pursue for cervical cancer. The patient may still be interested in having children, so treatments that will preserve the function of the uterus and cervix would be desired. The extent of the cancer will also be considered when deciding on a treatment plan.

- If childbearing is not a factor, a total **hysterectomy** along with removal of lymph nodes will be performed. Some surgeons can perform a procedure that only removes the cervix in patients who still wish to have children.
- **Radiation therapy** is usually performed to ensure destruction of cancer cells. When lymph nodes are involved, chemotherapy will also be performed.
- **Chemotherapy** can be done palliatively or when distant metastasis is involved.
- The best treatment is **screening** with regular Pap smears. The incidence of cervical cancer has decreased because of the increased awareness of the importance of early detection.

POSTOPERATIVE NURSING CARE FOR A HYSTERECTOMY

Postoperative assessment of the cancer patient who has undergone a **hysterectomy** includes assessment of vital signs and lung and bowel sounds. **Hemorrhage** is a postoperative risk factor and women who have undergone a vaginal hysterectomy are at a higher risk. Nursing staff should assess the incisional site for redness, warmth, edema, or drainage, and report any signs or symptoms of infection. Patients should be encouraged to cough and breathe deeply by splinting the abdomen with a pillow. Pain should be proactively managed. Intake and output should be accurately recorded, and fluid intake should be encouraged. **Deep vein thrombosis (DVT) prophylaxis** is critically important in patients who have undergone abdominal surgery. Patients are at a higher risk of developing a pulmonary embolus. The patient should be educated on perineal care. Patients who have undergone a hysterectomy may experience a negative self-concept and have misconceptions after their surgery. Nursing staff can help to clarify any misconceptions patients may have postoperatively through education and support.

OVARIAN CANCER TREATMENT OPTIONS

Treatment options for ovarian cancer include the following:

- Surgical removal of the ovaries, an **oophorectomy**, is necessary. In some cases, just the malignant tissue is removed from the ovary, but only if it is very localized and isolated. Surgery can also be helpful in determining the extent of metastatic lesions present in the pelvic and abdominal cavities.
- **Radiation therapy** can be done to treat metastatic lesions. This can cause permanent tissue damage with multiple side effects, though. It is possible for radioactive treatments to be inserted in the abdomen to deliver a steady dose of radiation therapy to metastatic lesions.
- **Chemotherapy** can also be given, but is usually used with an early diagnosis or palliatively in end-stage disease. Like the radioactive treatments, chemotherapy can also be given directly into the abdomen to provide more direct treatment to tumors. This also decreases the risk of side effects that are normally seen when chemotherapy medications are given orally or via IV.

UTERINE CANCER

Uterine cancer is primarily a late-onset, post-menopausal type of cancer. Most cases are endometrial adenocarcinoma, but about 1 in 20 cases involves uterine sarcomas. Endometrial cancers of the membrane lining the womb can be of either the hormonally dependent or independent type. Those that are hormonally dependent are characterized by hypertrophy or enlargement while those independent of hormonal control are associated with shrinking or atrophy of the endometrium. Cumulative exposure to estrogens, for example tamoxifen to treat breast cancer, is the greatest risk factor. Family history, obesity, and diabetes are other significant risk factors. Invasiveness and aggressiveness of uterine cancer is associated with more complex and atypical hyperplasia, certain subtypes (serous and clear cell carcinomas and uterine sarcomas), lack of progesterone or estrogen receptors, and overexpression of the p53 oncogene in the carcinomas. The main clinical presentation is abnormal uterine bleeding, which can also occur due to other conditions like fibroids or infection.

TESTICULAR CANCER

TREATMENT OPTIONS

A cure is usually possible with testicular cancer. Awareness of the disease has increased over the past several years, which has promoted self-examination and earlier treatment.

- Usually, the treatment of choice is an **orchiectomy** to remove the affected testicle. Depending on the severity of disease, lymph nodes from the pelvic cavity may also be removed for testing. If a single testicle is removed and the other is left and there is no presence of disease, the patient should not have any problems with normal sperm production in the future.
- **Radiation therapy** can be used to treat metastasis to the lungs. Permanent tissue damage can result from radiation treatments so the risks are weighed against the benefits.
- **Chemotherapy** may also be used with end-stage disease or a recurrent episode of testicular cancer. This is usually accomplished by using multiple drugs versus a single drug for treatment.

POSTOPERATIVE NURSING CARE FOR AN ORCHIECTOMY

Postoperative assessment of the cancer patient who has undergone an orchiectomy includes assessment of vital signs and lung and bowel sounds. Hemorrhage is a postoperative risk factor.

DVT prophylaxis should be initiated. The patient should be encouraged to cough and breathe deeply. The patient should be educated to avoid lifting and straining. **Hemodynamic status** should be carefully assessed postoperatively. The incision should be assessed for redness, warmth, edema, or drainage, and any signs or symptoms of infection reported. Pain should be proactively managed. Patients who have undergone an orchiectomy may experience a negative self-image. Discussions regarding body image concerns and sexuality should be encouraged. Patients who undergo more extensive surgery including bilateral orchiectomy with lymph node dissection are at a greater risk for sexual dysfunction. Patients may also have concerns regarding fertility. Patients should be educated on fertility-sparing measures prior to surgery as cryopreservation of sperm preoperatively is the most effective means of fertility preservation.

HEAD AND NECK CANCERS
MANAGEMENT

A primary consideration for management of early-stage head and neck cancers is preservation of functions like speech and swallowing if possible. Therefore, either external beam or brachytherapy radiation is often utilized. Otherwise, tailored site-specific surgical resection is used. With more advanced head and neck cancers, typical management is either surgery followed by radiotherapy or radiation along with chemotherapy. The latter approach has greater potential for organ preservation. Treatments for local or regional recurrences depend on whether the patient has received prior irradiation. If the patient has not been irradiated, radiation is given after resection or with chemotherapy. If the patient has received radiation, he or she may still be irradiated or given an implant along with surgery, if possible, or systemic chemotherapy. Palliation for very advanced cancers is usually chemotherapy, although radiation is sometimes used. All options have potential complications including potential nerve damage and loss of function with surgery, bone marrow suppression with chemotherapy, and a host of skin and tissue changes and functional losses with radiation.

POSTOPERATIVE NURSING CARE FOR AN OROPHARYNGEAL SURGERY

For patients with advanced laryngeal cancer, extensive glottic carcinomas, subglottic tumors, and advanced tumors of the base of the tongue that involve the larynx, a total **laryngectomy** may be indicated in conjunction with radiation therapy. Postoperatively, careful assessment of the patient's **airway** is critical. The patient should be closely observed for signs of respiratory distress. Suctioning may be necessary to help the patient clear secretions. The head of the bed should remain elevated to promote ventilation and decrease swelling. Tracheostomy care should be provided as needed to maintain patency of the stoma. Pain should be managed proactively and the patient should be placed on a bowel regimen to prevent constipation. The surgical site should be assessed for redness, warmth, or edema. Patient education regarding care of the tracheostomy should be completed early in the postoperative period to allow time for the patient to learn how to complete it independently. A dietitian should be involved with patients to ensure they are receiving the nutritional formula and number of calories that meet their needs.

CNS CANCERS

Central nervous system (CNS) cancers usually present as cognitive and personality changes, seizures, headaches, nausea and vomiting, or small lumps due to increased intracranial pressure, fluid buildup, and tissue destruction. The individual may have difficulty speaking or walking. If the patient has a tumor affecting the posterior fossa, he or she may have hydrocephalus (increased cerebrospinal fluid) due to compression of the fourth ventricle, which can result in a loss of the ability to control muscle movements. Loss of sensation or partial paralysis on one side of the body can be associated with brainstem gliomas. CNS cancers originating in the pineal gland region affect reflexes in the eye region. The best diagnostic imaging technique is MRI with gadolinium used as contrast, although others are used for various purposes. Management depends on the histologic type of the cancer. Surgical resection is usually the treatment of choice. Radiation is used as an adjunct for certain tumor types, particularly those of primitive or germ cell origin. Either option is appropriate for certain CNS tumors and chemotherapy is often used concurrently as well.

CARCINOMATOUS MENINGITIS

Any type of cancer cell can spread into the leptomeningeal space, the site of soft tissues surrounding the brain, causing **carcinomatous meningitis**. This diffusion of malignant cells can be caused by spread after surgical resection, hematogenous dissemination, or other contacts. These patients have advanced systemic malignancies and short survival times of a few weeks. Characteristic neurological signs occur with this dissemination of malignant cells into the leptomeningeal area, including double vision, hearing loss, difficulty swallowing, incontinence, back pain, headaches, and hydrocephalus. The cerebrospinal fluid is generally analyzed for cytology, cell counts, protein and glucose concentrations, and internal pressure. Cytological findings are the diagnostic tool of choice, but they have low predictive value. Radiographs may show hydrocephalus (increased fluid collection in areas of the brain) in the absence of a recognizable tumor mass. Imaging studies are generally inconclusive. The patient should be treated aggressively with radiotherapy and/or intrathecal chemotherapy using a ventricular catheter. Systemic administration of methotrexate has also been effective.

LIVER AND BILE DUCT CANCERS

About a million new **liver or hepatocellular cancer (HCC)** patients are identified yearly. Previous cirrhosis of the liver, usually caused by hepatitis B or C infection or alcohol consumption, is the main risk factor associated with development of liver cancer. **Gallbladder cancer** and cholangiocarcinoma (bile duct cancer) are much rarer than liver cancer. Most of these cancers are adenocarcinomas, which originate in glandular epithelia. Patients may be asymptomatic or exhibit jaundice, which is yellowing of the skin and other surfaces due to bile pigments in the skin. The best screening test for HCC is serum α-fetoprotein (AFP) levels. Imaging techniques, such as CT scans or MRI, and diagnostic tests for hepatitis B and C markers are generally done. AJCC staging confines T1 and T2 to single tumors without or with vascular invasion or small multiple tumors, T3 is larger multiple tumors or spread to a major vein, and T4 is dissemination to other organs or the peritoneum. Other neoplasms should be excluded on differential diagnosis. If possible, the affected organ should be completely removed surgically to increase chances of survival. Otherwise, the only recourse is the use of experimental protocols. The prognosis is relatively poor.

CARCINOMA OF THE PANCREAS

Generally, only up to about 15% of **pancreatic tumors** can be resected by pancreaticoduodenectomy (Whipple procedure) with adjuvant chemoradiation, a strategy increasing mean survival to about 18 months. Otherwise, most individuals with unresectable or metastatic disease can expect to live less than a year. Palliation strategies are employed to alleviate pain, jaundice, and/or gastric outlet obstruction. They include insertion of endoscopic or percutaneous transhepatic biliary stents, gastric or bile duct bypass operations, alcohol blockage of the celiac plexus, and chemoradiation. If metastases are present, chemotherapeutic agents are generally used to alleviate symptoms.

CANCER OF THE STOMACH

Cancer of the stomach is relatively common, with the predominant type being adenocarcinoma. Gastric cancers are staged using modalities like imaging of the upper gastrointestinal tract, endoscopy in conjunction with biopsy and ultrasonography, a liver profile, a chest radiograph, and CBCs. CT scan and laparoscopy are good adjuncts to determine the degree of extra gastric involvement. If gastric cancer is identified early (no positive nodes and only mucosal or submucosal involvement), the probability of cure through primarily surgical subtotal or total gastrectomy is extremely high. Chemotherapy and radiation have been used as adjuncts with mostly equivocal results. One study suggests a multimodality approach may significantly improve the outcome. Unfortunately, most cases are discovered at later stages. Locally advanced disease has been managed with a combination of external beam radiation and chemotherapy or surgery with limited success. Resection of part of the stomach or combination chemotherapy is sometimes used to palliate symptoms in advanced disease as well.

CANCER OF THE RECTUM

Rectal cancer is fairly common. It usually presents with rectal bleeding, changes in bowel habits, mucous in the stool, a feeling of fullness, and difficulty expelling feces. Staging is done by using rigid proctosigmoidoscopy in conjunction with rectal examination (pelvic or prostate assessment for women and men respectively). A colonoscopy or double barium enema, endorectal ultrasound, and other imaging studies using MRI and CT scans are performed. Many patients with rectal cancer also have colon cancer, and metastatic spread is usually to the liver, although other organs such as the lungs may be affected. CEA levels greater than 20 ng/mL can indicate metastases. PSA levels are measured in men as well. Other tumors and inflammatory processes are excluded by differential diagnosis. Most rectal tumors are treated by surgical resection even up to stage T3. Most node negative patients can be cured by surgery. Multimodal approaches have been tried as well.

KIDNEY, URETER, AND BLADDER CANCERS

The most frequent type of cancer of the kidney and ureter is **renal cell carcinoma (RCC),** a type of adenocarcinoma. There are several histologic types of RCC, which may be found together in these carcinomas. RCC is generally managed with a radical nephrectomy. Post-surgical adjuvant regimens with IL-2, interferon-α, thalidomide or other agents are under investigation.

The goals of **treatment for bladder cancer** are to remove the cancer and prevent metastasis, as well as maintain appropriate bladder function.

- Resection is frequently accomplished through a procedure called a **transurethral resection** (TUR). The tumor is usually burned electrically or with lasers in this procedure, but bleeding and healthy tissue damage can also occur.
- **Chemotherapy** is used by implanting the medications within the bladder to treat the tumor. Some of the common chemotherapy drugs used can cause a severe depression of the immune system.
- **Surgery** can be performed to remove the bladder and prostate and create a urinary diversion to be used for voiding. A **hysterectomy** is also performed in female patients. This surgery commonly causes sexual dysfunction.
- **Radiation** can also be performed to attempt destruction of the tumor cells. Damage can occur to healthy tissues as well, though. Radiation therapy is usually used when the bladder cancer is advanced.

POSTOPERATIVE NURSING CARE FOR A CYSTECTOMY

The standard treatment for bladder tumors that invade the muscle is surgical removal of the bladder by **radical cystectomy**. Postoperative nursing care includes assessment of vital signs and lung and bowel sounds. Urinary output should be closely monitored and maintained at a minimum of 30 mL/hour. The surgical site should be assessed for redness, warmth, edema, or drainage, and any signs or symptoms of infection reported. Signs of peritonitis related to an anastomotic leak include fever, leukocytosis, abdominal distension, and tenderness. The stoma should be assessed as well as the surrounding skin. Pain should be proactively managed. Patients who have undergone a cystectomy may experience a negative self-image. Patients should be encouraged to discuss their feelings regarding body image and sexuality. Patient education on cleansing and care of the stoma should be performed. Patients with a continent reservoir who will perform self-catheterization will need education on how to complete the catheterization.

SARCOMAS

Sarcomas are malignant tumors of mesodermal origin derived from connective tissue, bone, cartilage, or striated muscle. They can spread through invasion into nearby tissues or via the bloodstream. The majority of sarcomas diagnosed originate from soft tissue, and in some cases germline mutations appear to play a role in the development. Soft tissue sarcomas are managed by surgical resection with sufficient margin and usually radiation before or after surgery. Metastatic disease is treated with chemotherapy or, if the lungs are involved, pulmonary metastasectomy. Almost a quarter of new sarcoma cancers occur in the bone, with the vast majority of local occurrences in the extremities. These are usually treated successfully with limb-sparing procedures and customized reconstruction, including materials like implants.

MALIGNANCIES ASSOCIATED WITH HIV INFECTION

Infection with **HIV (usually HIV-1)** or human immunodeficiency virus has been found to increase the risk for development of non-Hodgkin lymphoma, Hodgkin disease, and Kaposi's sarcoma (KS). About half of HIV-positive patients who present with lymphomas are also infected with Epstein-Barr virus, and all of those who have Kaposi's sarcoma are positive for KS herpesvirus (KSHV). Kaposi's sarcoma affects the skin and other mucous membranes, and it usually presents as plaques, papules, or nodules on the lower limbs. Lymphomas have been previously discussed. CD4+ T-cell counts and HIV viral loads are measured for evaluation of both Kaposi's sarcoma and lymphoma associated with HIV. Biopsy and CT scans of the chest and abdominal region are usually done for KS patients. Management includes antiretroviral therapy to treat the HIV infection, other drugs for opportunistic infections (particularly for Pneumocystis), and systemic anthracyclines or paclitaxel. For lymphoma concurrent with HIV infection, antiretroviral drugs are used in conjunction with cytotoxic agents, hydration, and allopurinol.

Management of Metastases and Other Cancer Complications

BONE METASTASES

Most bone metastases develop in the axial skeleton, the bones that make up the vertebral column, skull, pelvis, and ribs, without significant lung involvement. The axial skeleton is rich in red bone marrow, and the slow-moving blood probably allows tumor cells to affix more readily. In children and adolescents, bones are primarily being built up, but in adults there is a constant remodeling cycle in which new bone is being formed or resorbed in response to osteoblasts or osteoclasts, respectively. The most important impact from the development of bone metastases is skeletal damage in response to the tumor, mediated by the osteoclasts in the presence of osteoblasts. Tumor cells also release a number of cytokines and growth factors that promote bone resorption either directly or through stimulation of immune cells. Parathyroid hormone related protein appears to play a role as well. Both lytic and sclerotic bone disturbances can be observed.

TECHNIQUES TO DISTINGUISH FROM OTHER SKELETAL DISORDERS

Other skeletal disorders can imitate bone metastases, including osteoporosis, degenerative diseases, Paget's disease, and bone fractures. On a plain **radiograph**, metastases favoring osteoclast overstimulation (typically from breast, lung, or GI cancer) show lytic areas; those arising from prostate cancer show sclerotic or hardened areas from bone growth with fibrous layers. In a bone scan, a radioactively-labeled compound with an affinity for calcium or hydroxyapatite in the bone is injected intravenously. A scan reveals patterns of blood flow and metabolic responses in the bone. CT scans or MRI can elucidate pathology when the scan is positive but the radiograph is normal.

BIOCHEMICAL MARKERS FOR BONE FORMATION AND RESORPTION

Measurable biochemical markers for bone formation include propeptide of type 1 procollagen (PICP), which is the antecedent to the main protein in bone called type 1 collagen, bone isoenzyme estimation related to alkaline phosphatase (ALP-BI), and serum osteocalcin (BGP) levels. Markers for bone resorption include serum and urine calcium concentrations, urinary hydroxyproline levels, concentrations of N- and C-terminal breakdown products of type 1 collagen (Ntx and Ctx), and the levels of compounds that crosslink collagen found in the urine. The latter crosslinking compounds include pyridinoline (PYD) and deoxypyridinoline (DPD). Sequential measurement of bone markers has been suggested as a means of detecting early bone metastases.

EVALUATION OF RESPONSE TO TREATMENTS

The response to management of bone metastases is evaluated in terms of relative bone repair and damage. Complete responses are rare. Plain radiographs are generally taken but are not particularly informative. When lytic-type metastases respond to treatment, they typically undergo sclerosis or harden. A characteristic *flare response* in which there is initial apparent deterioration followed by improvement is usually evidenced on bone scans. For the first few months after treatment, tracer uptake intensifies due to bone cell growth, and later uptake subsides on the scan when repair is complete. Sequential CT scans in which target metastatic sites are observed over time for changes are useful for evaluating treatment responses for lytic bone metastases. Interpretation of changes in sclerotic spots is difficult using any of these techniques.

USING TUMOR OR BIOCHEMICAL MARKERS TO ASSESS TREATMENT

Certain **tumor markers** have some utility in the assessment and management of malignancies and bear some correlation to associated metastases. They include carcinoembryonic antigen (CEA) and CA 15-3 for breast cancer and prostate specific antigen or PSA for prostate cancer. Calcium levels can be important predictors of treatment response, with a sharp decline in urinary levels indicative of effectiveness. The collagen crosslinkers PYD and DPD elevate significantly with metastatic progression. Serum calcium levels, urinary Ntx concentrations, and other biochemical markers of bone resorption tend to be higher if the metastasis is still progressing.

EXTERNAL BEAM RADIATION THERAPY AND TARGETED RADIOISOTOPE THERAPY

Local external beam radiation therapy palliates bone pain in the vast majority of patients. If there are numerous metastatic sites, then widefield irradiation of either the upper or lower body might be performed instead. This latter type, also called **hemibody irradiation**, is quite effective in relieving pain symptoms, but it induces GI problems later. Radioactively-labeled tracers that target absorption in specific sites are theoretically great tools for managing bone metastases. In this case, the **isotope** acts directly on the tumor cell. Radionuclides of the alpha- or beta-emitting type with long half-lives (such as 131-iodine or 89-strontium) are injected, and symptoms are relieved in most patients who concentrate the isotope in the desired area.

SYSTEMIC THERAPIES

The response to systemic agents such as bisphosphonates and calcitonin varies depending on the site of the primary tumor. For patients with metastases associated with primary breast carcinoma, treatment modalities can be either endocrine therapy or, in the case of aggressive disease, cytotoxic chemotherapy. Hormonal treatments with tamoxifen, aromatase inhibitors and/removal of the ovaries are considerably more effective in regressing tumors in hormone receptor positive patients. These receptors are estrogen and progesterone receptors, ER and PgR respectively. Prostate cancer patients are also managed with hormone therapy, in this case surgical castration or administration of anti-androgens or luteinizing hormone-releasing hormone (LHRH) agonists. Chemotherapeutic regimens with bone marrow-sparing agents are appropriate for some breast cancer patients, but are rarely used for prostate carcinoma. The most promising class of compounds for alleviation of bone pain and prevention of skeletal disease are bisphosphonates.

BISPHOSPHONATES

Bisphosphonates basis for utility is that they can induce apoptosis of osteoclasts, the cell type in bone associated with bone resorption. Bone pain associated with many tumor types can be relieved by intravenous administration of bisphosphonates. Some studies also suggest anti-tumor activity with use of these compounds. Most trials studying the effect of bisphosphonates, used in conjunction with other treatments in breast cancer patients, have employed intravenous pamidronate, and they indicate that it is effective in reducing skeletal morbidity. Bone resorption is disproportionately high in patients with multiple myeloma; thus, the infusion of pamidronate once a month is standard management practice. In men with prostate cancer, trials have generally not indicated any significant improvement with use of bisphosphonates, probably due the osteoblast origin of the lesions. Zoledronic acid is one of the most promising agents for prostate cancer, and has shown some promise for other cancers.

COMPLICATIONS

Cancer patients with metastatic bone lesions generally have the complication of bone pain, particularly back pain in conjunction with spinal instability. Pain relief for instable spines includes various stabilization procedures and percutaneous vertebroplasty, which is the introduction of an acrylic polymer into the vertebrae. Another frequent complication is hypercalcemia of malignancy, characterized by high serum calcium concentrations and loss of renal function. Bisphosphonates, in particular zoledronic acid, are used to manage acute episodes of this complication. Another quite critical complication can be spinal cord compression. Fractures are common problems, especially with lytic lesions. When these fractures occur in the ribs, other sequelae such as restrictive lung diseases can occur. Internal nailing or joint replacements in conjunction with other treatments are usually done to stabilize the fractures.

LIVER METASTASES

The major (often the only) site of metastases for some cancers is the liver, particularly for primary malignancies of gastrointestinal origin. Patients with melanoma and breast and lung carcinomas also frequently develop liver metastases. Imaging modalities are used to diagnose this liver involvement, especially computed tomography variations selecting for both soft tissues and abdominal structures. The best diagnostic variations are CT angiography or portography in which contrast is injected into either the hepatic or superior mesenteric arteries before imaging. Scans after later IV injection of iodine, which is picked up by the liver tissues but not the tumor cells, are also useful. T2-weighted MRI imaging is often used for detection of the irregularly shaped malignant lesions. Intraoperative ultrasonography and PET scans are other possible diagnostic tools. Hemangiomas, cysts, fatty infiltrates, and flow artifacts are all benign conditions that can be confused with liver metastases, without careful interpretation of these images. The laboratory test with the highest diagnostic value is CEA, while lactate dehydrogenase (LDH) is also a prognostic tool. The utility of other liver function tests is minimal.

HEPATIC RESECTION
PROGNOSIS, SURVIVAL RATES, AND PROBABILITY OF RECURRENCE

The significant parameters related to good prognosis after hepatic resection are:

- A tumor size of less than 5 cm
- Dukes stage B as opposed to stage C
- A disease-free interval of more than 2 years
- A larger resection margin
- A CEA value of less than 5 ng/mL

Most, but not all, clinical studies looking at staging of primary colorectal cancers (one of the primary malignancies often associated with liver metastases) also found that 5-year survival rates were significantly higher if the colorectal cancer was Dukes stage B and not stage C. Metastatic hepatic lesions recur in a significant number of patients after resections, regardless of whether the initial metastases were observed in the liver, elsewhere, or both. Additional surgical removal has been found to provide 3-year further survival rates of at least 33% without significant operative mortality.

ADJUVANT THERAPY AFTER HEPATIC RESECTION

Hepatic artery infusion (HAI) with chemotherapeutic agents after surgical resection of liver metastases has been found to increase the disease-free interval and survival time. These improvements are additive in relation to subsequent systemic administration of chemotherapeutic drugs. Generally, floxuridine (FUDR) (with or without dexamethasone) has been used for the HAI, and 5-fluorouracil, alone or in combination, has been the systemic agent. Other approaches like post-surgical adjuvant regional therapy or systemic administration of chemotherapeutic agents alone have been less well studied.

SYSTEMIC OR NEOADJUVANT CHEMOTHERAPEUTIC REGIMENS FOR LIVER METASTASES

The successful use of systemic chemotherapeutic regimens to treat liver metastases is highly correlated with the response to chemotherapy of the primary tumor. Nevertheless, quite a few studies have shown that once a malignancy has metastasized to the liver, chemotherapeutic drugs are less effective there than at soft tissue metastatic sites. Early introduction of systemic chemotherapy is suggested for patients with primary breast, colon, and gastric cancers with liver involvement. In general, combination therapies are more successful. Neoadjuvant therapy, in which the drugs are given before (or in this case sometimes in place of) surgical resection in order to reduce the tumor burden, has only been evaluated retrospectively, but it appears to be a useful tactic.

HEPATIC ARTERIAL INFUSIONS

Metastases frequently either begin in or are entirely confined to the liver. They have been carried there through the blood supply from the portal vein, but once in the liver the metastases are selectively infused by the hepatic artery. Some chemotherapeutic agents, in particular FUDR, are sequestered in the liver and can be administered locally at high dosages, without entering the general circulation, by hepatic arterial infusion (HAI). Currently, **HAI is usually done by surgically implanting a reservoir attached to a hepatic artery catheter**. The only significant toxicities with this approach have been gastritis, ulcers, and hepatic toxicities primarily affecting the bile duct. Laboratory measurements like SGOT and bilirubin are elevated in the latter case. Other complications, such as the formation of blood clots in arteries, are usually due to incorrect placement of the pump or failure to tie off branches of the gastroduodenal artery that supply organs like the pancreas or bile duct.

THERAPY

The majority of **efforts to decrease hepatic toxicity inherent with HAI** have been to use other drugs in conjunction with FUDR (in particular dexamethasone), to alternate administration of FUDR and 5-FU, or to mete out the FUDR according to the patient's circadian rhythm. The use of 5-FU for the HAI in conjunction with systemic leucovorin is another common approach. Response rates to hepatic arterial infusion therapy have been increased with **combination chemotherapeutic regimens**, but in general, toxicity has also been increased. HAI does not preclude development of extrahepatic metastases, which occur in up to 70% of patients, regardless of liver response. Studies using simultaneous therapies like intra-arterial and intravenous administration of FUDR to reduce extrahepatic involvement have not shown any substantial reduction in disease.

HEPATIC ARTERIAL LIGATION AND EMBOLIZATION

Hepatic arterial ligation (HAL) is the surgical tying of the hepatic artery in order to restrict the blood supply to the tumor, and thereby theoretically reduce the tumor burden. The technique is fairly effective for neuroendocrine tumors but not for less vascular tumor types such as those which commonly metastasize from the colon. Therefore, hepatic artery embolization (HAE) may be done alternatively; in this case, particles that cut off blood flow (such as microspheres) are instilled into the hepatic artery instead. The use of HAE with or without HAL is still controversial because it tends to produce untoward side effects, such as damage to other organs near the liver, blood clots in the lungs, liver function abnormalities, and renal insufficiency. HAE is most useful for management of the more vascular tumors, such as the aforementioned neuroendocrine tumors of the liver. A variation of HAE is chemoembolization in which drugs or radioisotopes are incorporated into the embolic agent.

WHOLE-LIVER IRRADIATION AND LOCALIZED RADIATION THERAPIES

The liver does not tolerate whole-liver irradiation well. When radiation dosages approach the 30 Gy range, the patient can develop complications (usually transient) induced by the radiation called "radiation-induced liver disease" or RILD. RILD is characterized by fluid accumulation in the absence of jaundice, liver enlargement, evidence of occlusion, and extremely elevated alkaline phosphatase levels. Therefore, if whole-liver irradiation is done, current dosages are usually smaller and combination regimens using radiosensitizing drugs, such as 5-FU or FUDR are generally utilized.

Several types of localized radiation therapies have been tried, including introduction of microspheres containing yttrium-90 into the hepatic artery, interstitial brachytherapy installed via laparotomy, careful external beam irradiation methods targeted through use of 3-D conformational techniques, and delivery of a large single bolus of irradiation to a small site.

ADDITIONAL MANAGEMENT MEASURES FOR LIVER METASTASES

Other techniques of management for liver metastases include:

- **Cryosurgery**: The use of very low temperatures to destroy cells, delivered using cryoprobes either during surgery or percutaneously and usually used in conjunction with other modalities
- **Heat therapies**: Two types generally used for smaller tumors
  - **Radiofrequency ablation**: Percutaneous placement of a tiny electrode inside the tumor to excite molecules and ultimately produce frictional heat and destroy cells
  - **Microwave coagulation**: The use of an external probe to produce microwaves, which shrinks the vascular bed and induces coagulation

136

- **Percutaneous ethanol injection (PEIT)**: The instillation of absolute ethanol directly into the tumor (using guiding ultrasound), which may be useful for small lesions but needs further documentation
- **Segregation of hepatic arteries and other local blood vessels** with clamps, followed by insertion of a catheter into the hepatic artery
- **Gene therapy**

PULMONARY METASTASIS

DIAGNOSIS

The primary location of metastases in patients with sarcoma is the lung, and pulmonary metastasis can also occur with other malignancies. Patients are usually asymptomatic, although some have coughs (possibly expelling blood) or vague chest pains. On traditional chest radiographs, a pulmonary metastasis is usually seen as a well confined nodule located in peripheral regions. Some lesions, such as those associated with squamous cell carcinomas, are cavitating in appearance; there may be air in the pleural cavity, and calcifications may be observed. CT scans are often used supplementally to look for pulmonary lesions, but this technique does not necessarily pick up more sites or differentiate well between malignant and benign processes. The utility of other imaging modalities, such as MRI or positron emission tomography with ^{18}F-flurodeoxyglucose, is still unsettled.

SURGICAL TREATMENT

If pulmonary metastases are unilateral, meaning they are found as a single lesion or only on one side of the lung, the **surgical approach** of choice is a posterolateral thoracotomy. The resection or metastasectomy is done by making an incision into the thorax, usually from the front into the fifth intercostal space. Another more controversial technique is video-assisted thoracoscopy (VATS); it is less painful for the patient but cannot pick up deep lesions well and is largely reserved at present for diagnosis or removal of a single metastasis. If bilateral disease (on both sides) of the lung is observed, there are several surgical techniques used. These include median sternotomy (an incision through the sternum), and several potential types of incisions through the thorax, variously called clamshell, sequential bilateral, and simultaneous bilateral thoracotomies. The preferred goal is to remove all metastases at once. Usually, the excision site is formed into a wedge with a stapling device before removal or electrocautery may be used.

PULMONARY METASTASECTOMY

PATIENTS WITH PRIMARY COLORECTAL CANCERS

Cancer patients whose primary tumor was colorectal often develop metastases, including metastatic lesions in the lung. About half of those with pulmonary metastases also have elevated levels of carcinoembryonic antigen. High serum CEA levels and the presence of multiple bilateral metastases are negative prognostic factors for the success of **pulmonary metastasectomy**. If the mediastinal or hilar lymph nodes are malignant, their dissection generally does not improve survival time. Nevertheless, pulmonary metastasectomy is still performed on many of these patients, although other approaches such as chemotherapy may be used. Concurrent resections of the liver, if involved, do not impact success of the pulmonary removal.

PATIENTS WITH PRIMARY BONE AND SOFT TISSUE SARCOMAS

Cancer patients presenting with primary bone and soft tissue sarcomas have a poor response to systemic agents and often develop metastases, especially in the lung(s). High grade undifferentiated sarcomas lead to lung metastases in the majority of patients. Here, the treatment of choice is definitely surgical resection. Lesions often return, but sequential resections are generally performed, and survival times are consequently increased. Five-year survival rates as high as 40% have been documented. Malignant hilar or mediastinal lymph nodes are rarely observed with bone and soft tissue sarcomas.

OTHER CANCER PATIENTS

Pulmonary metastasectomy may be done in for metastases associated with other primary cancer sites, including:

- **Melanoma**: With lung metastases found mostly in association with nodular or thick melanomas, resections improve survival, but the overall prognosis is poor.
- **Renal cell carcinoma**: Patients often develop distant metastases including in the lung(s); isolated resections in the lung dramatically increase survival rate, although frequent regional lymph node involvement indicates a poor prognosis.
- **Head and neck cancers**: These patients often develop primary lung tumors and/or metastases; surgical resection is the treatment of choice, and the prognosis is better for primary glandular tumors than those of squamous cell origin, as tumors of squamous cell origin often metastasize to the lung.
- **Breast carcinoma**: There is pulmonary involvement in up to a quarter of patients with metastases; resection is usually not indicated as the cancer is typically treated systemically.
- **Testicular and other germ cell cancers**: Pulmonary involvement can include up to half of these patients; there are excellent survival rates with the use of pulmonary resections.

MALIGNANT PLEURAL EFFUSION

The pleura is a thin transparent membrane lining the chest wall and the lungs that form a sac called the pleural space. This space contains fluid derived from the systemic blood supply; the purpose of the pleural fluid is to provide lubricated movement during respiration. Normally levels of pleural fluid are kept fairly constant at 7 mL per lung by assimilation of excess fluid into the capillaries and protein into the lymphatics. However, if this regulation is disrupted by the presence of malignancy, higher fluid levels can accumulate, causing a **pleural effusion**. An effusion involves excessive fluid in the pleural space due to factors such as increased pressure in the vessels, decreased pressure in the pleural space, depressed oncotic pressure (derived from plasma protein abnormalities), or increased permeability of the capillaries or lymphatics. Many conditions can cause this last feature, including increased permeability, malignancy, collagen vascular disorders, and infections. Fluid buildup can also be caused by depression of fluid removal as a result of mechanisms that constrict the lymphatics (including cytokine-mediated reactions, metastases, and damage after tumor treatments) or high systemic venous pressure.

> **Review Video: Pleural Effusions**
> Visit mometrix.com/academy and enter code: 145719

DIAGNOSIS AND EVALUATION

After congestive heart failure, malignancies are among the most common causes of pleural effusion, with the greatest number resulting from the presence of lung cancer. Primary breast carcinoma, lymphomas, and leukemias account for many effusions as well. Patients with pleural effusion experience shortness of breath (especially when prone), coughing, and chest or pleuritic pain. Their breath sounds are depressed or absent. Fluid buildup can be considerable, but it can be missed on normal chest radiographs unless both lateral and posteroanterior views are taken. **CT scans and ultrasounds** are useful adjuncts. Fluid is often withdrawn through a procedure called thoracentesis to determine whether the effusion has formed in loculi or cavities. In a cancer patient with pleural effusion, it is important to determine whether the effusion is a noninflammatory transudate or an exudate. An exudate is usually more serious, and it is derived from some active inflammatory or permeability problem.

EXUDATE

A pleural effusion categorized as an **exudate** is more critical to treat than one that is a transudate. Immediate appraisal of effusion samples may provide clues to its nature, as exudates are often purulent or bloody. Further, the ratio between pleural and serum cholesterol levels is at least 0.3 for exudative effusions (or a concentration >45 mg/dL by other criteria), while pleural LDH levels are in the high normal range (a ratio of pleural to serum >0.6), and protein in the pleural fluid is at least half the serum concentration or more than 2.9 grams per deciliter. Other diagnostic signs of exudative effusions are a pH of less than 7.3 as measured by blood gases, cytological studies indicative of malignancy, and elevated CEA levels.

EVALUATION OF EFFUSION OF ASSUMED MALIGNANT ORIGIN

Pleural effusions of assumed malignant origin are usually evaluated using **thoracoscopy**, or the insertion of an endoscope through an incision in the chest wall into an intercostal space. These thoracoscopies can be either medical or video-assisted (VATS). Medical thoracoscopy is generally performed by a pulmonologist who inserts a rigid scope into the pleural cavity while the patient is under conscious sedation and only local anesthesia. VATS is usually done by thoracic surgeons; the patient is given general anesthesia and ventilation, and there are various entry points. Other adjuncts may include the use of imaging procedures, such as chest X-rays, mammograms, or computed tomography scans, and cytology.

EFFUSION-TARGETED THERAPIES

In general, patients with larger pleural effusions have advanced stage cancers and will not respond well to systemic therapies. Their effusions are treated with **targeted therapies**:

- **Combination chemotherapeutic regimens** are useful if the primary tumor is a lymphoma or leukemia, and steroids are effective frontline medications for multiple myeloma patients.
- Some solid tumors (such as small cell lung carcinoma and tumors of germ cell origin) and their effusions respond well to **chemotherapy**.
- A major intervening modality targeted to the effusion itself is **therapeutic thoracentesis** in which large amounts of fluid are withdrawn, providing symptomatic relief. However, the cavity usually refills and dyspnea returns.
- Another technique, called **chemical pleurodesis**, introduces chemicals into the plural space that irritate the pleura while the effusion is simultaneously drained. With this technique, ultimately, the pleural surfaces fuse or sclerose but the exact mechanisms are unclear.
- Additional options include other surgical procedures, such as the creation of shunts, introduction of cytotoxic or other neoplastic agents into the pleural cavity, and the insertion of drainage catheters.

TALC AND OTHER SCLEROSING AGENTS

There are many agents that have been found to cause **pleurodesis**, or the adherence of the visceral and parietal layers of the pleural membrane. These chemicals essentially cause sclerosis of the membrane and include many cytotoxic drugs, inflammatory agents, coagulation factors, and irritants. The most commonly used sclerosing agent is **talc**, which is presented either through a chest tube as a saline slurry or blown into the cavity with a syringe or atomizer during thoracoscopic drainage. Talc induces pleurodesis at extremely high rates, regardless of the amount or method of introduction. The most serious possible complications are acute respiratory distress syndrome, inflammation of the lungs, and respiratory failure. Therefore, if talc is used, low doses (up to 5 milligrams) are recommended. **Bleomycin** is another sclerosing agent that is often used. Pleurodesis may also occur simply through mechanical means of irritation such as having a chest tube in place.

PERICARDIAL EFFUSIONS

The **pericardium** is a fibrous sac surrounding the heart and attached to major blood vessels. It normally contains a small amount of fluid whose dynamics are regulated by the same forces that regulate pleural fluid. Because the pericardial space is considerably smaller than the pleural space, any fluid changes can cause acute symptoms. These can include a rapid heart rate and palpitations, shortness of breath even when lying down, edema, cold extremities, and a protruding jugular vein. The effusion prevents the cardiac volume from changing, causing a weakening pulse on inspiration during measurement of blood pressure. **Pericardial effusions** can result from metastatic infiltration, but there are a wide variety of other causes including infections, cardiac diseases such as myocardial infarction, drug responses, and collagen vascular diseases.

DIAGNOSIS AND EVALUATION

The following are ways that pericardial effusions of malignant origin are diagnosed and evaluated:

- **Imaging modalities** (radiographs, CT scans, and MRI) are used to assess the degree of cardiac tamponade, or mechanical compression, caused by the effusion.
- **Electrocardiograms** are performed to identify masses in the heart.
- A procedure called **pericardiocentesis**, in which the pericardium is punctured and fluid is aspirated, is usually done.
- **Cytological studies, cell counts, and sometimes microbial cultures** are performed on the aspirated pericardial fluid; pericardiocentesis can also normalize fluid levels and provide symptomatic (but usually transient) relief.
- The rate of detection of malignant origin is low with cytology alone, but adjuncts like **biopsy** and an endoscopic technique called **pericardioscopy** can provide additional information.

MANAGEMENT

Systemic chemotherapeutic regimens are rarely used to manage pericardial effusions of malignant origin because of the critical nature of their presence. **Chemotherapy** has been utilized effectively in patients whose primary cancer is lymphoma, leukemia, a germ cell malignancy, or occasionally breast carcinoma. A **pericardiostomy**, in which a surgical opening for drainage is created percutaneously, is standard practice for other patients, and a variation using a balloon-dilating catheter is also promising. **Instillation of sclerosing agents** into the pericardium appears to control these effusions, similar to their utility in the management of pleural fluids; however, this technique may cause severe pain. Many pericardial effusions are managed surgically via a **subxiphoid pericardiostomy**, which involves the insertion of a more permanent chest tube for drainage and also creates irritation and promotes sclerosis. Most other surgical approaches offer no advantage over subxiphoid pericardiostomy.

MALIGNANT ASCITES
DIAGNOSIS AND EVALUATION

The sub-mesothelial lymphatic vessels are located within the peritoneal cavity lining the abdomen, and contribute to essential peritoneal fluid management. However, fluid can build up within the membranous peritoneal sac through dynamic processes similar to those observed with pleural or pericardial infusions. Here the fluid accumulation is called **ascites**, which in cancer patients is generally due to increased fluid creation. Cytokines contribute to most ascites production, in particular vascular epithelial growth factor (VEGF). Diagnostic symptoms include a distended abdomen, edema, GI problems, or dyspnea if the ascites is significant. Other diagnostic tools include ultrasound and physical examination; dull reflexes in the lower torso are indicative of malignant ascites. CT scans are useful for the identification of a primary malignancy or certain metastases in the presence of ascites. Fluid is withdrawn under local anesthesia and analyzed for cytology to identify malignant cells, cell counts, visual characteristics, the presence of albumin, and often tumor markers like CEA or CA-125. Milky-looking fluid termed chylous ascites can be due to either the presence of a tumor or cirrhosis. Ascites can be uniformly bloody or have high albumin levels when the underlying cause is malignancy.

MANAGEMENT OF FLUID BALANCE

Ascites fluid accumulation can be controlled somewhat by noninvasive measures, such as restriction of dietary sodium, limiting the use of intravenous hydration, and the administration of distal tubule diuretics. The latter strategy is controversial because the mechanism of ascites production generally does not involve pressure gradients and because volume depletion and electrolyte abnormalities can result from diuretic use. Repeated paracentesis or needle aspiration of fluid provides transient relief. Other effective and longer-lasting approaches include peritoneovenous shunting between the thoracic and abdominal cavities, external insertion of drainage catheters for repeated use, intraperitoneal injection of chemotherapeutic drugs or biological response modifiers, and surgical peritonectomy. Surgical approaches have not been well studied.

Treatment Administration

PROFESSIONAL QUALIFICATIONS NEEDED TO ADMINISTER CHEMOTHERAPY

For a nurse to be qualified to administer chemotherapy, the following is required:

- Current license as a registered nurse
- Certification in CPR
- Skill in intravenous therapy
- Educational preparation and demonstrated knowledge in all areas related to neoplastic drugs, including preparation, disposition, elimination, and interactions
- Demonstrated knowledge of preparation of medication errors and skill of drug administration
- Ongoing acquisition of updated information and verification of continuing knowledge and skills
- Policies and procedures that govern specific actions for chemotherapy administration

SELECTION AND PREPARATION OF INSERTION SITE

Generally, the central vein of choice for the insertion of vascular access devices is the **subclavian vein**. Nevertheless, the internal jugular vein offers many advantages over the subclavian, including an easier and more direct placement of the guiding wire and less possibility of puncturing the subclavian artery or introducing air or blood into the thorax. The carotid artery can also be perforated during insertion into the internal jugular vein, but this is easily managed with the application of pressure. Maintenance of a sterile environment during insertion is paramount. For surgically implanted devices, this means the use of sterile fields, protective clothing, and cleaning the patient's skin with a topical antimicrobial agent (preferably chlorhexidine). Other decisions to consider before insertion include the placement site for the catheter tip (the intersection between the subclavian vein and the right atrium is recommended) and whether to use antibiotic-saturated catheters or guiding aids such as ultrasound.

The **process for site selection** is as follows:

1. The site selection should begin with a critical assessment of all available veins of the patient.
2. All equipment for venipuncture should be assembled before any attempt is made.
3. During vein selection, avoid any arm with known or proven compromised circulation.
4. To preserve venous integrity over time the nurse should begin distally and alternate venipuncture sites.
5. If there is no site available by observation, use of a tourniquet is permissible.
6. A cannula should be selected that is appropriate for both the length of the therapy and the patient's available veins.
7. If the drug is to be given via a freely-running side arm, the dressing should not hinder visualization.
8. When injecting a vesicant do not use an infusion pump.
9. If a drug in combination is known to be associated with rapid onset of nausea and vomiting, it is given <u>last</u>.
10. The entire course of the vein should be visible during the injection or infusion.
11. A vesicant should not be injected distal to a previous site.
12. Vesicant agents should not be infused as a mini-infusion or continuous infusion into a peripheral vein.

SELDINGER INSERTION TECHNIQUE

During any insertion technique, the patient is monitored by electrocardiograph and oxygen monitors. In the **Seldinger technique**, which may be used to access either the subclavian or jugular vein, the patient's clavicle bones are first opened up by the placement of a towel under the vertebral column. The patient sits on a table tilted 45 degrees with his or her legs hanging over the edge. A mild tranquilizer such as benzodiazepine is given by IV through a peripherally inserted line. The skin area is treated with both an antimicrobial agent and the anesthetic 1% lidocaine, which is also delivered by IV to the insertion tract. If the subclavian vein is being utilized, the long insertion needle is introduced gradually underneath the clavicle just above the sternal notch until a little negative pressure is felt and blood is drawn. Then the syringe is detached and replaced by the catheter or guiding wire. The tip should be placed just above the intersection of the subclavian vein and the right atrium, which can be documented by x-ray or fluoroscopy. If the right internal jugular vein is used, then the needle is inserted a few centimeters above the right clavicle near the sternocleidomastoid muscle.

INSERTION OF PERMANENT SILASTIC CATHETERS

Silastic catheters are made of a rubber-like silicone and generally used for permanent insertions such as continuous infusion therapy. The Hickman catheter is a common example of this type. Two small 1 cm incisions are made. The first is cut at the normal access site but antibiotics are initially introduced before catheter insertion. The second incision is made inferior to the other, on the chest near the fourth or fifth intercostal space. The catheter is pulled up to the upper incision site using a suture through a tunnel starting at the lower slit. It is then held in place and trimmed to the needed length for positioning. The catheter is then inserted into the sheath of another piece of equipment called an introducer kit (which is later removed) for positioning. Other neck veins can be used by changing the placement of the tunnel.

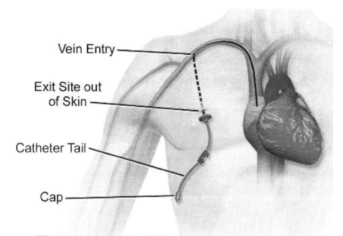

Tunneled Central Venous Access Device

INSERTION OF IMPLANTED INJECTION PORTS

When injection ports are surgically implanted, two incisions are made in sites similar to those used for Silastic catheters. However, in this case, the lower incision is larger, about 3 cm, and a suture is used to tunnel downward to the lower site before the port is attached and a subcutaneous pocket is cut. The port is sutured in place into the pocket, and the site is covered with an impermeable dressing. The upper incision is typically made into the subclavian vein. After implantation, intermittent infusions can be injected into the port and led through the tunnel into the subclavian vein.

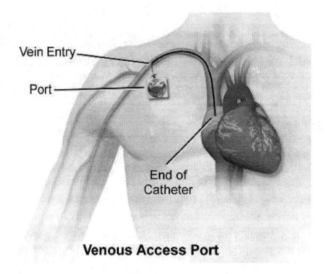

Venous Access Port

PRETREATMENT CONSIDERATIONS

Prior to cancer treatment, the following factors must be considered:

- Make sure the patient is completely informed about the treatment plan.
- Make sure there is a **signed** informed consent form.
- Check the drug dosage against the physician's order.
- Check the patient's last laboratory results.
- If the WBC is low, calculate the AGC (absolute granulocyte count): [(% of neutrophils) + bands X total WBC = AGC].
- Consider the way each drug is metabolized and eliminated. If an impaired organ is involved, toxicity may result.
- Consider any pretreatment antiemetics, hydration, or measures to eliminate resulting alopecia.
- Make sure that emergency equipment is near at hand to counter any allergic reaction or extravasation of drug or vesicant.
- Ensure adequate lighting and patient comfort.
- Review the patient's entire medication history (for incompatibilities, interactions, and toxicities).

VASCULAR ACCESS DEVICES

Vascular access devices are used to enter the central vascular system where there is greater blood flow. The major devices are listed below. They can be used for infusion of nutrients, chemotherapeutic drugs, or for blood drawing:

- **Percutaneous central lines** are laced just under the skin and led through a wire into either the subclavian, internal jugular, or femoral vein. They are for short-range use, as they are prone to infections.
- **Surgically tunneled central lines** are longer lines that are channeled subcutaneously into central veins, usually surgically implanted. These lines are for long-term use (up to several months) and are held in place by a Dacron cuff that promotes scar-cuff tissue adhesion, lessening the chance of infection.
- **Surgically implanted infusion ports** are connected to internal catheters leading to either the subclavian or internal jugular vein and are surgically implanted. The reservoir has a resealing cap and can be accessed externally with a special needle for adding agents or obtaining blood withdrawal without appreciable infection or leakage.
- **Peripherally inserted central catheters (PICC)** are placed in a peripheral vein (brachial, cephalic, or antecubital) and then led into the subclavian or other central vein; one of the easiest access methods, but may induce thrombosis
- **Short-term venous catheters** can be inserted into peripheral or central veins and are generally utilized for less than two weeks. These can be used for multiple medications, including chemotherapy or total parenteral nutrition (TPN). Because they are more often used in smaller peripheral veins, damage to these vessels can occur with infusion of more caustic agents.
- **Long-term venous catheters** are inserted when infusion is necessary for longer than two weeks. These are generally inserted into larger veins, such as the jugular or either vena cava, and are used for infusion of medications and TPN. A sterile dressing is required and the patient can frequently go home with these lines to administer medications on their own.
- **Arterial catheters** are also used when arterial access is necessary. These are frequently used when high doses of chemotherapeutic medications must be given.

INFUSION SYSTEMS

The type of infusion systems utilized in cancer treatment administration is dependent on the type of treatment:

- **Large volume infusion systems** are used for infusions that will take longer to administer. They can be electric IV pumps or pumps that control multiple infusions at once. These are used primarily when infusing blood or various medications, including antibiotics and chemotherapy.
- **Small volume infusion devices** are used for medications that will be infused quickly. These are frequently used for antibiotics and may be electronically controlled or pressure released.
- **Patient-controlled infusions** give the patient the ability to administer their own medication. These are frequently used for IV analgesics through patient-controlled analgesic pumps (PCA pumps). The IV pump is programmed to allow only a certain amount of medication to be delivered with each dose with a total amount to be given within a certain time period. This prevents any problems with overdosing. The pump can also be set with a basal rate which automatically provides a specific amount of medication to be delivered.

> **Review Video: Calculating IV Drip Rates**
> Visit mometrix.com/academy and enter code: 396112

GUIDELINES FOR ADMINISTERING ANTINEOPLASTIC AGENTS

Guidelines for administering antineoplastic agents are specific to the route of administration:

- **Oral**: Emphasize the importance of complying with the prescribed schedule. Plan for drugs with emetic potential to be taken with meals and for drugs that require hydration to be taken early in the day.
- **Subcutaneous or intramuscular**: Demonstrate and require the patient to perform a return demonstration to ensure the patient understands if doing self-injections. Encourage rotation of injection sites.
- **Topical**: Cover surface with a thin film of the medication. Instruct the patient to wear loose-fitting cotton clothing. Wear gloves and wash hands thoroughly.
- **Intra-arterial**: This method requires catheter placement in an artery near the tumor. Administer in a heparinized solution through an infusion pump. Monitor the patient throughout treatment. Instruct the patient and the significant other on the use of the pump if medication is to be given at home.
- **Intracavitary**: Instill the drug into the bladder through a catheter or chest tube into the pleural cavity. Follow instructions carefully.
- **Intraperitoneal**: Place the drug into the abdominal cavity through an implantable port or external suprapubic catheter. Warm the solution to body temperature before giving it to the patient.
- **Intrathecal**: Reconstitute all medications with preservative free sterile normal saline or sterile water. (Usually, a physician administers intrathecal drugs.)
- **Intravenous**: Drugs may be given through intravenous catheters or peripheral vein access. Follow the institution guidelines for administration of drugs.

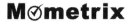

ACUTE AND LATE-ONSET COMPLICATIONS OF VASCULAR ACCESS DEVICES

When vascular access devices are inserted, the most common **acute complications** are the introduction of air into the pleural cavity, excessive bleeding, and the possibility of cardiac dysrhythmias. Bleeding in association with low platelet levels is a frequent complication for cancer patients. Introduction of air into the pleural space, or pneumothorax, can be controlled with good technique. Transient cardiac dysrhythmias generally occur when the device comes in contact with the right atrium, disturbing conduction pathways.

Delayed complications include development of infections, blood clots, leaking of solution in surrounding subcutaneous tissue (extravasation), and compression of the line between the clavicle and first rib, which interrupts flow.

INFECTION AND THROMBUS

Development of **infections**, particularly with coagulase-negative staphylococci, is the primary late-onset complication of catheter use. Diagnosis usually involves microbial cultures of both the adjacent skin and the blood. The risk of infection is greatest for non-tunneled central venous access devices (particularly those with multiple lumens), which can be removed and replaced. Tunneled central lines and implanted infusion ports are less likely to become infected. However, as they are much more difficult to detach, removal is usually only done when there is sepsis or infection related to the tunnel or port.

Blood clots or **thrombi** tend to develop in central access devices. They are usually discovered when routine heparinized saline flushing is noted to be difficult. The presence of any thrombus further disposes the patient to infection, especially at the site of insertion. If there is evidence of a fibrin sheath on the tip (gravity flow shown but no blood return) or an occluded catheter (no flow in either direction), declotting with urokinase or tissue plasminogen activator is indicated. Otherwise, removal or repositioning is usually done.

MANAGEMENT OF CATHETER-RELATED CLOTS

Initially, a **chest radiograph** is taken to identify the location of the clot. **Gravity flow tests** are then performed. These involve comparing the flow of normal saline connected to the catheter from above and below to identify positional or blood return problems. Catheters that have been positioned incorrectly will show gravity flow differences upon moving and generally need to be replaced, but some can be repositioned. For example, a transverse catheter that crosses over into the opposite subclavian space can be dragged down into the correct spot. If transient arrhythmias occur during any right atrium contact, gravity flow may be intermittent as well. Again, the catheter can probably be pulled down into proper position in the subclavian vein. Gravity flow abnormalities are not observed if the thrombus is located in a major vessel, but unilateral edema is seen instead. These cases require a hematology consult.